Exercise and Sport in Diabetes

Second Edition

Diabetes

in Practice

Other titles in the Wiley Diabetes in Practice Series

Obesity and Diabetes
Edited by Anthony Barnett and Sudhesh Kumar
0470848987

Prevention of Type 2 Diabetes
Edited by Manfred Ganz
0470857331

Diabetes: Chronic Complications Second Edition
Edited by Ken Shaw and Michael Cummings
0470865972

The Metabolic Syndrome
Edited by Christopher Byrne and Sarah Wild
0470025115

Psychology in Diabetes Care Second Edition
Edited by Frank J. Snoek and T. Chas Skinner
0470023848

Diabetic Cardiology
Edited by B. Miles Fisher and John McMurray
0470862041

Diabetic Nephropathy
Edited by Christoph Hasslacher
0471489921

The Foot in Diabetes Third Edition
Edited by A. J. M. Boulton, Henry Connor and P. R. Cavanagh
0471489743

Nutritional Management of Diabetes Mellitus
Edited by Gary Frost, Anne Dornhorst and Robert Moses
0471497517

Hypoglycaemia in Clinical Diabetes
Edited by Brian M. Frier and B. Miles Fisher
0471982644

Diabetes in Pregnancy: An International Approach to Diagnosis and Management
Edited by Anne Dornhorst and David R. Hadden
047196204X

Childhood and Adolescent Diabetes
Edited by Simon Court and Bill Lamb
0471970034

Exercise and Sport in Diabetes

Second Edition

Editor

Dinesh Nagi

Edna Coates Diabetes and Endocrine Unit, Pinderfields Hospital, Mid Yorkshire NHS Trust, Aberford Road, Wakefield, UK

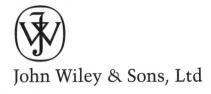

John Wiley & Sons, Ltd

Other Wiley Editorial Offices

John Wiley & Sons Inc., 111 River Street, Hoboken, NJ 07030, USA

Jossey-Bass, 989 Market Street, San Francisco, CA 94103-1741, USA

Wiley-VCH Verlag GmbH, Boschstr. 12, D-69469 Weinheim, Germany

John Wiley & Sons Australia Ltd, 33 Park Road, Milton, Queensland 4064, Australia

John Wiley & Sons (Asia) Pte Ltd, 2 Clementi Loop #02-01, Jin Xing Distripark, Singapore 129809

John Wiley & Sons Canada Ltd, 6045 Freemont Blvd, Mississauga, Ontario, Canada L5R 4J3

Wiley also publishes its books in a variety of electronic formats. Some content that appears in print may not
be available in electronic books.

Library of Congress Cataloging-in-Publication Data

Exercise and sport in diabetes/editor, Dinesh Nagi – 2nd ed.
     p. ; cm.
   Includes bibliographical references and index.
   ISBN-13 978-0-470-02206-X (alk. paper)
   ISBN-10 0-470-02206-X (alk. paper)
   1. Diabetes–Exercise therapy.   2. Sports–Physiological aspects.
   3. Exercise–Physiological aspects. I. Nagi, Dinesh.
   [DNLM: 1. Diabetes Mellitus–metabolism. 2. Exercise–physiology. WK 810 E96 2005]
RC661.E94E94 2005
616.4′62062–dc22   2005029358

British Library Cataloguing in Publication Data

A catalogue record for this book is available from the British Library

ISBN-13 978-0-470-02206-1 (H/B)   ISBN-10 0-470-02206-X (H/B)

Typeset in 10.5/13pt Times by Thomson Digital
Printed and bound in Great Britain by Antony Rowe Ltd., Chippenham, Wilts
This book is printed on acid-free paper responsibly manufactured from sustainable forestry
in which at least two trees are planted for each one used for paper production.

Contents

Foreword to the First Edition

Anyone setting out to write a book on diabetes and exercise must come to grips with the fact that the risks and benefits are very different for the two types. The editors are to be congratulated for having got the balance right.

Let us consider the type 2 diabetes problem first. In 1997, it was calculated that it affected 124 million people in the world, and this is expected to rise to 221 million by 2010.[1] The numbers are startling but the conclusion, that this epidemic is due to a deficiency of physical exercise, is not new. In the *Medical Annual* of 1897, the Birmingham physician, Robert Saundby, wrote that, 'Diabetes is undoubtedly rare among people who lead a laborious life in the open air, while it prevails chiefly with those who spend most of their time in sedentary indoor occupations', and the next year he added, 'There is no doubt that diabetes must be regarded as one of the penalties of advanced civilisation'. The real question is what can we do about it. Thomas McKeown[2] and others have suggested that we should stop research into the minutiae of genetics and put all our money into preventive medicine and public health, and it is certainly true that effective action will only come in the public health arena with government support. It has also been suggested that we should return to palaeolithic patterns of food and physical activity,[3] and we know, from O'Dea's classical experiment in returning acculturated aborigines to a traditional lifestyle, that this would work.[4] It is, however, difficult to imagine people willingly dispensing with their cars and convenience food. For the next few decades, I think the only practical solution is for the problem to be tackled on a local basis by diabetes care teams, which is why they need to read this book.

The problem in type 1 diabetes is entirely different. I agree with Dr Grimm (Chapter 2) that exercise is not a tool for improving blood glucose control, and that its benefits relate to the cardiovascular system (unproven) and to bolstering self esteem by allowing participation in a more normal lifestyle. Hopefully diabetes care teams who have read this book will help their patients avoid the experience of the tennis player, Billy Talbert.[5] He explained that, when entering his first tennis tournament in 1932 at age 16:

> I had to go on and explain about the diabetes. It took some talking on my part to persuade her that I was fit to enter her husband's tournament and even then she kept eyeing me as if she expected me to drop at any moment. Her husband relieved her – and discomfited me – by promising to have a doctor at the courts.

What is really useful about this book is the wealth of practical advice, which is available in one place for the first time – previously one had to scour journal articles and back copies of *Balance* to find it. Will your patient on insulin be able to box? (no, and a jolly good thing too!) or bobsleigh down the Cresta Run? (again, no). Most other reasonable opportunities for physical recreation are allowed, and the authors explain in admirable detail how diabetic patients should prepare themselves. This is an excellent book which should be on the shelves in every diabetic clinic.

ROBERT TATTERSALL,
Special Professor of Metabolic Medicine,
University of Nottingham, Nottingham, UK

References

1. Amos AF, McCarty DJ, Zimmet P. The rising global burden of diabetes and its complications: estimates and projections to the year 2010. *Diab Med* 1997; **14**: S7–S85.
2. McKeown T. *The Origins of Human Disease*. Oxford: Blackwell Scientific, 1988.
3. Eaton SB, Shostak M, Konner M. *The Palaeolithic Prescription: a Program of Diet and Exercise and a Design for Living*. New York: Harper and Row, 1988.
4. O'Dea K. Marked improvement in carbohydrate and lipid metabolism in diabetic Australian Aborigines after temporary reversion to traditional lifestyle. *Diabetes* 1984; **33**: 596–603.
5. Talbert WF, Sharnick J. *Playing for Life*. Boston, MA: Little Brown, 1958.

Preface to the First Edition

Exercise, sport and physical activity pose a number of problems for professionals involved in the care of people with diabetes. On the one hand, there are increased numbers of people with type 1 diabetes. Their disease management may not be improved by playing sport and taking exercise, but it is entirely appropriate that they should be helped to take part in any sports that they may wish, in order to live life to the full. Health professionals need to be well informed to help them to do this while experiencing as little disruption as possible to daily life, and maintaining optimal levels of diabetic control to minimize the risk of complications.

These problems are entirely different from those encountered in the management of people with type 2 diabetes. We believe that a global epidemic of type 2 diabetes has begun, which will prove to be one of the biggest health challenges of the twenty-first century. The global prevalence of type 2 diabetes will have doubled in the decade 1990–2000 to an estimated 160 million, and the social and economic burdens of this will be enormous. Developing countries are being particularly affected and the costs of chronic microvascular and macrovascular complications are likely to be devastating. Various factors probably contribute to the current epidemic, and are the subject of considerable debate. Genetic, intrauterine and neonatal factors almost certainly have major effects, but the overwhelming importance of environmental factors such as age, obesity and physical inactivity cannot be denied. Obesity and physical inactivity are inextricably linked and are both potentially reversible and preventable by appropriate interventions.

There is evidence to suggest that the inexorable year-on-year rise in the prevalence of obesity in developed countries is not due to an overall increase in calorie intake but is more likely to be due to a decline in physical activity. This leads us to believe that type 2 diabetes should be regarded as a deficiency state, with the deficiency being physical activity.

The challenge to those of us involved in diabetes care in the twenty- first century will be to devise effective strategies to promote increased activity and physical fitness at the level of communities, as well as at the individual level. Interventions at individual level will have to be targeted at those with risk factors such as family history, ethnicity, gestational diabetes, obesity, hypertension and impaired glucose tolerance.

We hope that this book will provide arguments to support the need for increased resources to help diabetes teams tackle the lifestyle problems of people with type 2 diabetes. We hope also that it will aid the health professional faced with the need to provide people with type 1 or 2 diabetes detailed advice to help them exercise safely and with maximum enjoyment.

DINESH NAGI,
Edna Coates Diabetes and Endocrine Unit,
Mid-Yorkshire NHS Trust, Wakefield, UK

Foreword to the Second Edition

Although I have been a medical practitioner since 1984, my experience of diabetic management was very limited until 1997 when my husband, Steven Redgrave, was diagnosed with diabetes at the age of 35 years. His immediate reaction was one of devastation: why me? why now? it's not fair! He, like many others, had heard of the complications of diabetes and everyone he talked with seemed to have a nightmare to tell. He felt he was going to have to accept that this condition would finally prevent him from continuing to train. His life would never be the same again.

I was, at the time, the Chief Medical Officer for GB Rowing, confronted by a newly diagnosed diabetic asking questions about his future in sport, together with his coach and crewmates. I felt, whatever the final outcome, it was wrong to give in to the label of diabetes without trying. I searched for information or case studies that might help and for individuals who could offer advice – very little was available either in print or via the internet. It rapidly became apparent that there was no easy answer.

It was only by trial and error and with the help of a diabetologist prepared to challenge conventional diabetic management that a regimen was established which eventually culminated in Olympic gold in Sydney.

I cannot say it was easy, but the experience demonstrated to me, and hopefully this will become clear to anybody about to read this book, that diabetes should not be used as a reason to prevent somebody from exercising. Diabetes is just another variable that needs to be allowed for when writing an exercise programme. The diabetic needs to be safe when taking exercise and certain guidelines need to be followed, as laid out clearly in the text of this book.

It saddens me that diabetes today is still a condition that controls peoples lives. With modern insulins and multiple methods of administration, surely this no longer needs to be the case and all diabetics should be allowed to control their condition.

Exercise cannot be used to control blood sugar levels in type 1 diabetics but it plays an important role in reducing the insulin requirement of the individual and in their wellbeing.

Exercise can be used to control blood sugar levels in the type 2 diabetic and allows them more flexibility in their dietary control.

This book is a valuable resource for anyone advising a person with diabetes who engages in exercise and sport for it dispels common myths and allows the diabetic the same choices in life as the non-diabetic.

I only wish it had been available in 1997!

ANN REDGRAVE,
August 2005

Preface to the Second Edition

When the Publisher John Wiley approached Professor Bill Burr and myself to compile the first edition of this book in 1998, the need to produce a revised second edition never crossed our minds. However, since the first edition was published, there have been significant advances in our knowledge about the role of exercise in the prevention, as well as clinical management of, diabetes. These scientific advances have meant that the role of exercise in the prevention and management of diabetes is even more important than before. I have been asked on numerous occasions by Diabetes Teams in the UK to speak about exercise and sports in Type 1 and Type 2 diabetes, which highlighted to me the enormous interest in this topic and also the need for training for health professionals. There is certainly a growing realisation among Specialist Diabetes Teams that they have to address the needs of individuals with diabetes who wish to undertake sports and physical activity.

Since the publication of the UK's National Service Framework for Diabetes in 2002, there is a clear responsibility for the Primary Care Trusts to develop and implement strategies to prevent Type 2 diabetes. There have also been many campaigns, both locally and nationally, to move the population toward adopting a healthy lifestyle, e.g. the five-a-day programme (which encourages people to eat five units of fruit and/or vegetables each day). There is a need for public health workers to take a lead in this area to implement such programmes throughout the population. The physical activity level of the whole population needs to change and that can be achieved only by targeting the younger population at school. There is good evidence that people who are active when young stay active later in life as adults.

This second edition of the book contains three new chapters covering nutrition and diet in sports and exercise, the role of physical activity in the prevention of Type 2 diabetes and insulin pump therapy and exercise. These chapters describe the new evidence on the prevention of diabetes and also acknowledge the increasing popularity of Insulin pump therapy in the UK and elsewhere.

I hope that the second edition will be a significant advance over the first and will prove equally popular. I would like to extend special thanks to my senior co-editor on the first edition, Professor Bill Burr, who provided me with encouragement and inspiration to complete the revisions for this new edition. I hope that the book will be a useful resource for health care professionals and patients, who continue to tackle admirably the challenges posed by the burden of diabetes.

DINESH NAGI,
May 2005

Acknowledgement

I would like to sincerely acknowledge the tremendous help from Karen Bambrook for secretarial assistance in the preparation and proof reading of this book. Her generous and ever smiling support made the task so much easier and enjoyable.

List of Contributors

Bill Burr

The Department for NHS Postgraduate Medical and Dental Education, NHS Executive Nothern and Yorkshire, University of Leeds, Willow Terrace Road, Leeds LS2 9JT, UK

Alan Connacher

Perth Royal Infirmary, Perth, Scotland, UK

Sandra Dudley

Diabetes Centre, Harrogate District Hospital, Harrogate HG2 7SX, UK

Jean-Jacques Grimm

2 rue du Moulin, 2740 Moutier, Switzerland

Peter Hammond

Diabetes Centre, Harrogate District Hospital, Harrogate HG2 7SX, UK

Elaine Hibbert-Jones

Department of Nutritions and Dietetics, Royal Gwenth Hospital, Newport, South Wales NP20 2UB, UK

Alison Kirk

Institute of Sport and Exercise, University of Dundee, Old Hawkhill, Dundee DD1 4HN, UK

Elizabeth Marsden

School of Education, University of Paisley, University Campus Ayr, Beech Grove, Ayr KA8 0SR, UK

Dinesh Nagi

Edna Coates Diabetes and Endocrine Unit, Pinderfields Hospital, Mid Yorkshire NHS Trust, Aberford Road, Wakefield WF1 4DG, UK

Ray Newton

Nirewells Hospital, Dundee, Scotland, UK

Gill Regan

Department of Nutritions and Dietetics, Chief Royal Gwenth Hospital, Newport, NP20 2UB, South Wales, UK

Mark Sherlock

Department of Diabetes, Beaumont Hospital, PO Box 1297, Beaumont Road, Dublin 9, Ireland

Diarmuid Smith

Department of Diabetes, Beaumont Hospital, PO Box 1297, Beaumont Road, Dublin 9, Ireland

Chris Thompson

Department of Diabetes, Beaumont Hospital, PO Box 1297, Beaumont Road, Dublin 9, Ireland

Clyde Williams

School of Sport and Exercise Sciences, Loughborough University, Ashby Road, Leicester LE11 3TU, UK

1

Physiological Responses to Exercise

Clyde Williams

1.1 Introduction

Exercise presents a challenge to human physiology in general and to muscle metabolism in particular. How we meet these challenges depends on the exercise intensity, its duration, our fitness and our nutritional status. The aim of this chapter is to present an overview of the physiological responses to exercise which support muscle metabolism. The descriptions of carbohydrate metabolism during exercise and recovery are based on studies in non-diabetic, active individuals. The ways in which exercise affects carbohydrate metabolism in people with diabetes are discussed in Chapters 2 and 5, and in earlier reviews on this topic.[1,2]

1.2 Maximal Exercise

How we cope with exercise depends on several factors, central to which is our capacity to deliver adequate amounts of oxygen to our working muscles in order to prevent premature fatigue.

As we walk, cycle or run faster, there is a parallel increase in oxygen consumption (VO_2) due to aerobic metabolism, which is related to exercise intensity. This linear relationship between aerobic metabolism and exercise intensity holds true for most forms of physical activity.

Oxygen uptake continues to increase with exercise intensity until the maximum rate of oxygen consumption is reached ($VO_{2\ max}$). Exercise can be continued at a

Exercise and Sport in Diabetes, 2nd Edition   Edited by Dinesh Nagi
© 2005 John Wiley & Sons, Ltd.

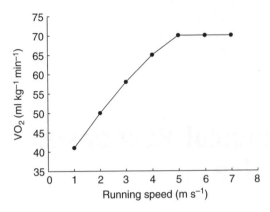

Figure 1.1   Schematic representations (based on actual data) of the relationship between the oxygen cost ($ml\,kg^{-1}\,min^{-1}$) of running on a level treadmill and running speed ($m\,s^{-1}$) during the assessment of an athlete's maximum oxygen uptake (VO_{2max})

higher intensity for a short while, without any further increase in oxygen uptake (Figure 1.1).

Maximum oxygen uptake is usually determined during exercise on a treadmill or cycle ergometer. Exercise intensity is increased step by step, either with short breaks between each stage or continuously to the point where the subject fatigues. There are field tests that can be used to estimate VO_{2max}, which do not require extensive and expensive laboratory equipment. One such method is a multistage shuttle running test which requires only a tape recorder and a 20 m space to perform the running test.[3] It is a test which is acceptable for untrained and trained people and requires little skill to perform and evaluate.

The size of an individual's VO_{2max} is determined by several factors, the most prominent of which are age, sex, height, weight, habitual level of physical activity and inherited factors. The genetic contribution to the physical size of an individual, including the cardiovascular system, reflected by VO_{2max}, is relatively large.[4]

However, most people who increase their habitual level of physical activity or undertake a training programme do not get even close to their genetic limit for VO_{2max}. It is only endurance athletes who have trained for many years who might get close to the genetic limit for their already high VO_{2max} values. Nevertheless, the amount of physical work that we can accomplish is largely dictated by the size of our VO_{2max} value. This relationship is certainly true for runners competing in long-distance races.[5,6] Elite endurance athletes can increase their oxygen uptake from resting values of $0.25\,l\,min^{-1}$ to peak values of $5.0\,l\,min^{-1}$ during maximum exercise lasting 2–3 minutes.

The key elements in the oxygen transport system are described by the Fick equation (see Table 1.1). Resting values for cardiac output, arteriovenous oxygen difference and oxygen uptake are similar for sedentary and well-trained indivi-

Table 1.1 The Fick equation

Fick equation
VO_2 = heart rate × stroke volume × arterio-venous oxygen difference
Rest
$0.25 \text{ l min}^{-1} (VO_2) = 5.0 \text{ l min}^{-1} (Q) \times 50 \text{ ml l}^{-1} (\text{A-v } O_2)$
Maximal exercise
Athletes: $5.0 \text{ l min}^{-1} (VO_{2max} = 30 \text{ l min}^{-1} [Q(max)] \times 166 \text{ ml l}^{-1}(\text{A-v } O_2)$
Active: $3.0 \text{ l min}^{-1} (VO_{2max} = 22 \text{ l min}^{-1} [Q(max)] \times 136 \text{ ml l}^{-1} (\text{A-v } O_2)$

duals. However, well trained athletes have maximum cardiac outputs in excess of 30 l min^{-1},[7] which allows them to increase their oxygen consumption by 20-fold above resting values. In comparison, active but not well-trained individuals can achieve a 12-fold increase in their oxygen uptake values during maximum exercise.

Maximum oxygen uptake varies with age, reaching a peak in the second decade of life and decreasing thereafter.[8] The rate of decline in VO_{2max} is greatest in those people who take little daily exercise and least in those who maintain a good level of physical activity throughout their lives.[8]

1.3 Submaximal Exercise

The physiological responses to submaximal exercise are not simply proportional to, for example, walking, running, cycling or swimming speeds, but to the relative exercise intensity.

The relative exercise intensity is defined as the oxygen cost of an activity expressed as a percentage of the individual's maximum oxygen uptake ($\%VO_{2max}$). The physiological responses to exercise, such as heart rate, temperature regulation and the proportion of fat and carbohydrate oxidized is proportional to the relative exercise intensity rather than the external intensity, e.g. running speed.

1.4 Endurance Training

Training improves oxygen delivery by increasing stroke volume (the amount of blood pumped with each heartbeat). This, in turn, increases maximum cardiac output without major changes in maximum heart rate, which remains unchanged or may even decrease. Training also increases the absolute amount of haemoglobin in the red blood cells carried in the blood (but not the concentration). Therefore it is not unusual for endurance athletes to have haemoglobin concentrations at the lower end of the normal range.[9] The apparent reduction in haemoglobin concentration with training is a consequence of a relatively greater increase in plasma volume than haemoglobin content.[10]

Training also increases the capillary density around individual muscle fibres, and so the delivery of oxygen to muscle becomes more efficient.[11] An increase in the mitochondrial density in muscle enables greater oxygen extraction during exercise, and increases the endurance capacity of an individual during submaximal exercise, without producing changes in maximum oxygen uptake. A contributory factor to the improved exercise tolerance is an increased capacity of trained muscle to extract oxygen from blood, which allows a decreased skeletal muscle blood flow during submaximal exercise.[12,13] This cardiovascular response to exercise, along with an increase in the aerobic metabolism of fatty acids for energy provision, and hence reduction in the formation of lactic acid, explains the improvements in exercise capacity after training. The increased aerobic metabolism of fatty acids reduces the demand on the limited glycogen stores and so delays the depletion of muscle glycogen.

Endurance-trained individuals have higher resting concentrations of muscle glycogen than untrained individuals.[14] The reason for this difference is not simply the higher proportion of carbohydrate consumed daily by endurance-trained individuals. Exercise stimulates the release of glucose transporter proteins from their storage sites within muscle to the membrane, where they help accelerate the transport of glucose into the muscle cell.[15] These GLUT 4 transporter proteins increase with training such that endurance-trained people have a larger complement than untrained people. Frequent low-intensity exercise not only increases GLUT 4 protein activity but also improves glucose tolerance.[16] However, the activity of the GLUT 4 transporter proteins appears to decrease quite markedly after a couple of days of inactivity.[17] This evidence suggests that exercise must be undertaken frequently if it is to be used to successfully manage type 2 diabetes (see review for recommendations[18]).

1.5 Muscle Fibre Composition

Skeletal muscles contain two main types of muscle fibres: the fast-contracting, fast-fatiguing fibres (type II) and the slow-contracting, slow-fatiguing fibres (type I). The rapidly contracting type II fibres generate the energy source, adenosine triphosphate (ATP), mainly by the breakdown of their glycogen stores (glycogenolysis). In addition to the rapid formation of ATP, they also produce lactic acid, or more correctly lactate and hydrogen ions. The accumulation of hydrogen ions in type II muscle fibres contributes to the onset of fatigue during sprinting. Training improves the aerobic capacity of these fibres, such that oxidative metabolism of glycogen makes a greater contribution to the production of ATP.

In contrast, the slow-contracting, slow-fatiguing type I fibres generate ATP by the oxidative metabolism of fatty acids, glucose and glycogen. The larger oxidative capacity of these fibres is the result of their greater mitochondrial density and better oxygen utilization than the type II fibres. The skeletal muscles of elite marathon runners contain more type I fibres than type II fibres and the converse is true for top-class sprinters.[19] The marathon runner who has only a small percentage of type II fibres may, of course, be beaten in a sprint to the finishing line by a competitor with a greater proportion of type II fibres.

During exercise of increasing intensity, the type I fibres are recruited first, followed by type II fibres. This conclusion has been drawn from histochemical examination of the glycogen depletion patterns in cross-sections of active muscle fibres.[20,21] Athletes who undertake training which is mainly of low intensity and long duration will not fully recruit, and hence train, their type II fibres. Sprinting recruits both populations of fibres because a large muscle mass is needed to generate high speeds. However, one of the limitations to maximum sprint speed is the slower speeds of type I muscle fibres. Nevertheless, the power developed during sprinting would be significantly less if only a proportion of the muscle mass was recruited. The question of whether or not fibre type conversion can occur in response to training has been examined for at least three decades. The general view is that adaptation of fibre types does occur, but the evidence from studies on human muscle is not as strong as that from animal studies (for review see Astrand, et al.[22] pp. 47–67).

1.6 Muscle Metabolism During Exercise

Both the respiratory and cardiovascular systems act in concert to provide working muscles with an adequate supply of oxygen for aerobic metabolism. Within the muscle cells, mitochondria produce ATP for contractile activity between the neighbouring elements, actin and myosin. In addition, the resting requirements of all cells are sustained by the continual provision of ATP, reflected by the resting metabolic rate. Oxygen plays its important role during the final step in aerobic metabolism. The stepwise degradation of the metabolites of fat and carbohydrate that enter the mitochondria releases hydrogen ions and, following subsequent coupling reactions, electrons from these metabolites are transported along an 'electron transport chain'. The final step in this complex process is the acceptance of these electrons by the available oxygen. The presence of oxygen as the terminal electron acceptor in the mitochondria allows the whole process of oxidative phosphorylation to flow successfully. The net outcome is that the adenosine diphosphate molecules (ADP) that were produced as a result of the energy yielding degradation of ATP are converted back to the much needed ATP. Some ATP is also generated by the phosphorylation of ADP from phosphocreatine (PCr). The resting muscle has about five times more PCr than ATP and so this important high-energy store acts as an energy buffer during the onset of exercise, when the rate of ATP resynthesis from glycogen and fatty acids is too slow to cover the energy expenditure of the working muscles. The first few steps in the degradation of muscle glycogen to produce ATP do not require oxygen and so are described as anaerobic glycogenolysis. Glycogenolysis provides some ATP rapidly, but only for a short time.

1.7   Anaerobic and Lactate Thresholds

The accumulation of lactate in the blood during submaximal exercise has been interpreted as an indication of an inadequate oxygen supply, and so there is a need for anaerobic glycogenolysis to contribute to ATP production.[23] The lactate and hydrogen ions diffuse into the venous circulation where the hydrogen ions are buffered by plasma bicarbonate. As a result of this 'bicarbonate reaction', there is an increase in carbon dioxide production which stimulates a rise in pulmonary ventilation.[24,25] This change in the rate of pulmonary ventilation has been proposed as a method of detecting the 'anaerobic threshold' or ventilatory threshold,[23] which may also correlate with a rise in blood lactate.[26,27]

Not everyone supports the concept of an anaerobic or ventilatory threshold. Lactate production occurs in skeletal muscle under fully aerobic conditions,[28,29] and this supports the view that lactate accumulation during exercise simply reflects an increased contribution of glycogenolysis to ATP production, rather than an inadequate supply of oxygen. However, a simple description of the anaerobic or lactate threshold is as follows: during exercise of increasing intensity, a point is reached where the aerobic provision of ATP is no longer sufficient to cover the demands of working muscles and so the anaerobic production of ATP increases to complement the existing oxidative production of ATP.

Rather than attempt to detect the precise lactate thresholds of an individual as part of a routine fitness assessment, lactate reference values are often used. For example, a blood lactate concentration of $4 \, \mathrm{mmol \, l^{-1}}$ has been described as the 'onset of blood lactate accumulation' (OBLA). This particular concentration represents, for many individuals, the beginning of a steep rise in blood lactate during exercise of increasing intensity.[30] It has been proposed that the 'aerobic' and 'anaerobic' thresholds occur at blood lactate concentrations of around 2 and $4 \, \mathrm{mmol \, l^{-1}}$ respectively.[31] Even though this is an over-simplification, these lactate concentrations provide useful reference points for the routine physiological assessment of the training status of sportsmen and women.[32]

For example, an analysis of poor exercise tolerance of an individual should consider whether or not the activity level is above or below the individual's anaerobic or lactate thresholds. Fatigue will occur earlier in those people who have low anaerobic thresholds than for those who have higher anaerobic thresholds.[33] The anaerobic or lactate threshold values of active people are usually expressed as a percentage of their $VO_{2 \, max}$,[34] and are calculated, for instance, during submaximal treadmill running. Subjecting less active people, such as those recovering from illness, to heavy exercise as a means of determining their VO_{2max} is unacceptable. However, their functional capacity can be assessed by determining, for example, the walking speed at which their blood lactate reaches a concentration of $2 \, mmol \, l^{-1}$. Monitoring this value during rehabilitation provides an objective way of following the increasing fitness of patients receiving treatment. The anaerobic or lactate threshold has proved to be a useful way of assessing the functional capacity (training status) of a person independently of their VO_{2max}.[34] The concept has been extended to the measurement of a 'maximum lactate steady state' as a more informative method of assessing training status and adaptations to training, i.e. endurance capacity. The rationale offered is that the maximum lactate steady state represents the balance between lactate appearance and disappearance from the blood, i.e. reflecting production and utilization.[35] However, this is a much more time-demanding assessment procedure than is the lactate threshold and so the method used is usually dictated by how the information is to be used. For example, the maximum lactate steady state may be the preferred method in research studies on training-induced adaptations in metabolism, whereas the lactate threshold often provides sufficient information for a routine fitness test on athletes.

During our daily round of activities, whether they are part of work or recreation, there are only a few occasions when the contribution of glycogenolysis to energy production is greater than the contribution from aerobic metabolism of fatty acids. Running for a bus, or participation in sports such as rugby, hockey, tennis or squash, requires maximum activity for no more than a few seconds. Under these circumstances, about half the ATP is provided by the phosphorylation of ADP by PCr, and the other half is contributed by glycogenolysis.[36] Even so, the contribution of anaerobic ATP production to overall energy production during participation in these multiple-sprint sports is relatively small compared with the contribution from aerobic metabolism. This is because the brief periods of maximum exercise, essential as they are, are punctuated by longer periods of submaximal activity such as walking, running or resting.

Aerobic metabolism of fatty acids and glucose, and breakdown of liver and muscle glycogen, supports energy production during rest and during exercise. As submaximal exercise continues, there is an ever-increasing contribution of fatty acids to muscle metabolism which coincides with a decrease in the glycogen stores in liver and active skeletal muscles. This shift in substrate metabolism is clearly illustrated during a treadmill marathon race (Figure 1.2).

As can be seen in Figure 1.3, carbohydrate oxidation decreases as the race continues, whereas fat oxidation increases. At about 35 km, fat and carbohydrate oxidation make equal contributions to energy metabolism, and racing speed is reduced (Williams, unpublished data). The reduction in running speed may be a consequence of an inability of the carbohydrate stores to continue to fuel ATP production at the rate required to maintain the initial running speed. The point in the race at which runners are forced to reduce their running speed has been described as 'hitting the wall' (see Figure 1.2).

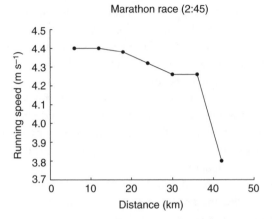

Figure 1.2   Running speeds of an experience marathon runner during a treadmill marathon (42.2 km), during which the runner set his own speed in order to achieve as fast a time as possible for this simulated race

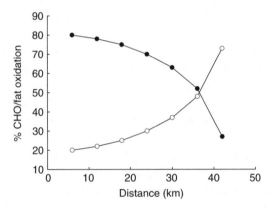

Figure 1.3   Relative contributions of carbohydrate (●) and fat (○) to energy metabolism during a treadmill marathon race

1.8   Fatigue and Carbohydrate Metabolism

As the glycogen stores are gradually used up during prolonged exercise, ATP resynthesis cannot keep pace with ATP demands within each of the active muscle fibres. Even with a contribution from intramuscular triglycerides, the high rate of ATP turnover during heavy exercise can be sustained only for as long as there is a sufficient supply of glycogen. Liver glycogen contributes to muscle metabolism via the provision of blood glucose but the delivery of this substrate is insufficient to replace the dwindling glycogen stores. When skeletal muscle glycogen concentrations reach critically low values, then exercise intensity cannot be maintained. Fatigue, under these circumstances, is clearly associated with the depletion of muscle glycogen stores. To combat this, it is not surprising that dietary manipulations have been developed to increase the body's carbohydrate stores in preparation for prolonged exercise, as well as to delay the depletion of muscle glycogen stores during prolonged exercise.

Helge *et al.* in 1996 [37] investigated the effects of high-fat and high-carbohydrate diets on endurance capacity during cycling to exhaustion. The subjects ate a diet which provided them with either 62 per cent of their daily energy intake from fat or 65 per cent from carbohydrates. They continued training for 7 weeks in total, and were tested after 4 and 7 weeks.

The endurance capacity of the group on a high-carbohydrate diet was significantly greater (102 min) than that of the group on the high-fat diet (62 min). In order to check that the greater endurance capacity of the subjects in the high-carbohydrate group was not simply the result of the preceding few days on a high-carbohydrate diet, the subjects in the high-fat diet group were switched to a high-carbohydrate diet for a week and both groups tested again. After a week on a high-carbohydrate diet the group who trained on the high-fat diet improved their cycling endurance capacity from 62 to 77 min, however, the group trained on the high-carbohydrate diet did not improve their endurance capacity beyond 102 min. One of the puzzling results of this study was the higher muscle glycogen concentrations of the group that trained on a high-fat diet prior to the exercise test at the end of the last week of training when all subjects consumed a high-carbohydrate diet. In spite of the higher pre-exercise muscle glycogen concentrations, their exercise time to exhaustion was significantly less than that of the group that trained on the high-carbohydrate diet. The authors suggest that training on the high-fat diet had failed to produce the adaptations that would have allowed these subjects to use the increased stores of glycogen during exercise.[37]

In a more recent series of studies on the potential benefits of high-fat diets, Burke and colleagues examined the influence of 5 days on either a high-fat or -carbohydrate diet that was followed by a rest day on a high-carbohydrate diet. On the seventh day the subjects cycled for 2 h at 50% VO_{2max} and concluded with a 'time-trial'.[38–40] Although there was an increase in fat oxidation during the prolonged period of submaximal cycling, even following a day on a high-carbohydrate diet, there were no differences in the time trial performances. Even if there are some benefits to be gained from a high-fat diet before exercise, the long-term disadvantages to the health of the individual must be weighed against possible short-term gains in endurance performance.

1.9 Carbohydrate Nutrition and Exercise

In developed countries, carbohydrates provide between 40 and 50 per cent of the daily energy intake of the population, whereas in developing countries carbohydrates contribute significantly more to daily energy intake.[41] Sedentary people who become active tend to increase their daily carbohydrate intake.[42] Sportsmen and women consume more carbohydrate than the population at large,[43] but even they may not eat enough to replace the carbohydrate used during daily training or competition.[44-46]

Athletes undertaking heavy daily training over prolonged periods benefit from a carbohydrate intake of between 60 and 70 per cent of their daily energy intake.[44] Most sportspeople obtain between 50 and 60 per cent of their daily energy intake from carbohydrates and adopt nutritional strategies to achieve high carbohydrate stores before and after heavy exercise or competition.

Dietary carbohydrate loading

In preparation for competition, most athletes taper their training in the week leading up to the event. Eating more carbohydrate during the 3–4 days before the competition is sufficient to increase muscle and liver glycogen stores to levels which are above normal values.[47] The recommended amount of carbohydrate is about 600 g a day (based on studies only in men). This amount of carbohydrate is clearly too great for women because it would account for almost the whole of their daily energy intake. A more helpful recommendation is one which is based on body mass, for example, $8-10 \, \text{g kg}^{-1}$ body mass per day for the 3–4 days before competition.

Dietary carbohydrate loading before cycling to exhaustion improves endurance capacity when compared with performances after a mixed diet. Early studies on carbohydrate loading reported improvements of 50 per cent in cycling time to exhaustion,[48] and the benefits of carbohydrate loading on endurance capacity during cycling have been confirmed repeatedly.[49] There have been relatively few studies on the effect of a high-carbohydrate diet on running performance, but Goforth and colleagues were amongst the first to report an improvement in endurance capacity of runners (9 per cent) after carbohydrate loading.[50] Improvements in endurance running capacity of about 25 per cent were also reported for male and female runners when they consumed a high-carbohydrate diet during the 3 days before a series of treadmill runs to exhaustion. One group supplemented their diet with simple carbohydrates (confectionery), and another group supplemented their diet with complex carbohydrates (pasta, potatoes and rice); the type of carbohydrate used had no influence on the subsequent improvement in endurance running capacity. Simply increasing energy intake in the form of additional protein and fat did not result in an improvement in endurance running capacity of a third group, confirming the importance of carbohydrate intake for improved performance.[51]

Competitors in a 30 km cross-country race clearly benefited from dietary carbohydrate loading during the 3–4 days leading up to this endurance competition. Ten runners completed the cross-country course on two occasions separated by 3 weeks.[52] On one occasion, five of the 10 runners ran the race after carbohydrate loading, while the others maintained their normal mixed diets. On the second occasion the runners swapped dietary preparations and were paid to match or improve on their performance times for the first race. All the runners improved their times for the 30 km following preparation on the high-carbohydrate diet (135 vs 143 min). This is probably the most informative study published on the influence of carbohydrate loading on running performance because not only was the study conducted as part of a real competition, but also muscle biopsy samples were obtained from the runners before and after both races.

The high-carbohydrate diet for 3 days before the race significantly increased the pre-competition muscle glycogen stores. Furthermore, the carbohydrate-loaded runners completed the race in shorter times and without such a pronounced reduction in muscle glycogen as in the race preceded by the mixed diet. It is clear from this and later studies that the size of the carbohydrate stores alone will not dictate the outcome of an endurance race. Pre-race muscle glycogen stores must be sufficient to meet the demands placed on them by the endurance race; however, the benefits of carbohydrate stores in excess of this amount have not been established. Although absolute proof is lacking, the current practice is to raise carbohydrate stores as high as possible, within the constraints of time, training and dietary preparation. Other than a slight gain in body mass, there appear to be no disadvantages to dietary carbohydrate loading.

In races over shorter distances, high pre-competition muscle glycogen concentrations do not appear to improve performance. For example, there were no differences in performance times for a 20.9 km race, on an indoor 200 m track, when well-trained runners consumed either a mixed diet or a high-carbohydrate diet 3–4 days before the race.[53]

In contrast, starting exercise with a less than adequate glycogen store will significantly reduce exercise capacity, as has been demonstrated in laboratory studies.[48,54] In real competitions, such as in a soccer match, those players who began the game with low muscle glycogen concentrations ran less than the rest of the team throughout the match.[55]

Most of the studies on the influences of dietary carbohydrate loading on exercise capacity have used men as subjects and some studies have failed to show the same benefits for women. Females use more fat for energy metabolism during sub-maximal exercise than males and the extent to which they are able to load their muscle glycogen stores may be somewhat less than has been reported for men.[56–58]

Pre-exercise meals

Eating before competition presents a problem for many people because they feel uncomfortable when they exercise shortly after a meal. The standard advice offered is to try to eat a high-carbohydrate meal, which is easy to digest, about 3 h before exercise. However, the description of carbohydrates as either simple or complex is an inadequate way of classifying them, because not all carbohydrates produce the same metabolic response. A more informative way of classifying carbohydrates is based on the degree to which they raise blood glucose concentrations. Carbohydrates which produce a large increase in blood glucose concentration, in response to a standard amount of carbohydrate (50 g), are classified as having a high glycaemic index (GI).[59] Table 1.2 presents a selection of foods and their glycaemic indices.[60] The metabolic responses during exercise are influenced by the glycaemic indices of the carbohydrates in the preceding meals, and so the choice of carbohydrate in pre-competition meals could have an effect on performance.

Some of the early studies on the glycaemic and insulinogenic responses to high-GI and low-GI carbohydrate foods reported only minimal changes in glucose and insulin concentrations following the consumption of low-GI foods.[62] The main reason for these responses is that they used single foods rather than a mixture of

Table 1.2 Glycaemic indices of common foods

Breads and grains		*Fruits*		Milk, full fat	27
Waffle	76	Watermelon	72	Milk, skimmed	32
Doughnut	76	Pineapple	66		
Bagel	72	Raisins	64	*Snacks*	
Wheat bread, white	70	Banana	53	Rice cakes	82
Bread, wholewheat	69	Grapes	52	Jelly beans	80
Cornmeal	68	Orange	43	Graham crackers	74
Bran muffin	60	Pear	36	Corn chips	73
Rice, wheat	56	Apple	36	Life savers	70
Rice, instant	91			Angel food cake	67
Rice, brown	55	*Starchy vegetables*		Wheat crackers	67
Rice, bulgur	48	Potatoes, baked	83	Popcorn	55
Spaghetti, white	41	Potatoes, instant	83	Oatmeal cookies	55
Spaghetti, wholewheat	37	Potatoes, mashed	73	Potato chips	54
Wheat kernels	41	Carrots	71	Chocolate	49
Barley	25	Sweet potatoes	54	Banana cake	47
		Green peas	48	Peanuts	14
Cereals					
Rice Krispies	82	*Legumes*		*Sugars*	
Grape Nuts Flakes	80	Baked beans	48	Honey	73
Corn Flakes	77	Chick peas	33	Sucrose	65
Cheerios	74	Butter beans	31	Lactose	46
Shredded Wheat	69	Lentils	29	Fructose	23
Grape Nuts	67	Kidney beans	27		
Life	66	Soy beans	18	*Beverages*	
Oatmeal	61			Soft drinks	68
All Bran	42	*Dairy*		Orange juice	57
		Ice cream	61	Apple juice	41
		Yoghurt, sweetened	33		

In the above table foods are listed from highest to lowest glycaemic index within each category. Glycaemic index was calculated using glucose as the reference with an index of 100.[60,61]

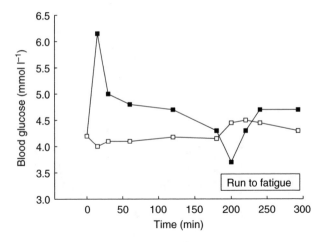

Figure 1.4 Blood glucose concentrations (mmol l^{-1}) of eight recreational runners before and after a high-GI (■) and low-GI (□) carbohydrate breakfast and during treadmill running to fatigue (the breakfast provided 2 g CHO kg^{-1} body mass; GI values for the high-GI and low-GI breakfasts were 74 and 26, respectively (adapted from Wee et al.[65]))

foods that are found in everyday meals. For example, when a group of runners ate a low-GI meal that contained lentils before exercise there was hardly any change in their blood glucose and insulin concentrations during the postprandial period. This suggests that very little carbohydrate is absorbed during a short postprandial period and so it may make little contribution to the carbohydrate metabolism during subsequent exercise (see Figures 1.4–1.6). This was confirmed in a

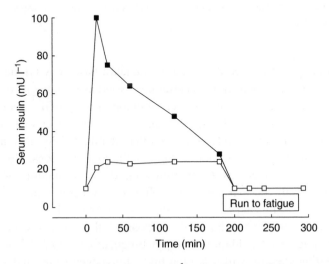

Figure 1.5 Serum insulin concentrations (mU l^{-1}) of eight recreational runners before and after a high-GI (■) and low-GI (□) carbohydrate breakfast and during treadmill running to fatigue (the breakfast provided 2 g CHO kg^{-1} body mass; GI values for the high-GI and low-GI breakfasts were 74 and 26, respectively (adapted from Wee et al.[65]))

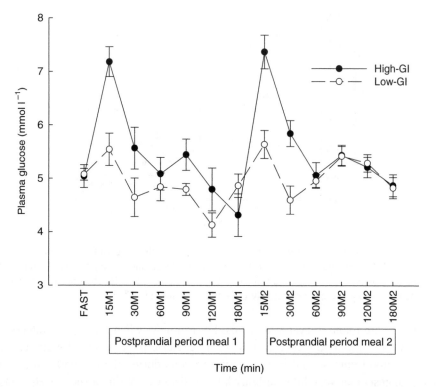

Figure 1.6 Plasma glucose concentrations of seven male recreational runners following the ingestion of a high-GI (•) and a low-GI (o) breakfast and a high-GI and low-GI lunch (all meals provided 2g CHO kg^{-1} body mass; GI values for the high-GI and low-GI breakfasts were 77 and 44, respectively, and for the high-GI and low-GI lunches were 73 and 38, respectively (adapted from Stevenson et al.[64]))

subsequent study that showed that 3 h after the lentil-based low-GI meal there was no change in muscle glycogen concentrations, whereas muscle glycogen concentration increased by 15 per cent after consumption of a high-GI carbohydrate pre-exercise meal.[63] Eating low-GI meals that contain carbohydrate foods that are more palatable and more widely consumed than lentils will result in a significant increase in both blood glucose and serum insulin concentrations. However, these changes are not as great as those following the consumption of a high-GI carbohydrate meal. Furthermore, the blunted glycaemic and insulinogenic responses to a low-GI meal persist even after a second meal (Figures 1.6 and 1.7).[64]

This reduction in the insulinogenic response following a low-GI meal may increase the rate of fat oxidation during subsequent exercise.[62,66] Increasing fat oxidation during exercise will spare the limited glycogen stores and so provide a clear advantage during endurance activities. Some, [62,67,68] but not all, studies [65,69] have concluded that endurance exercise capacity is improved following the consumption of low-GI carbohydrate meals.

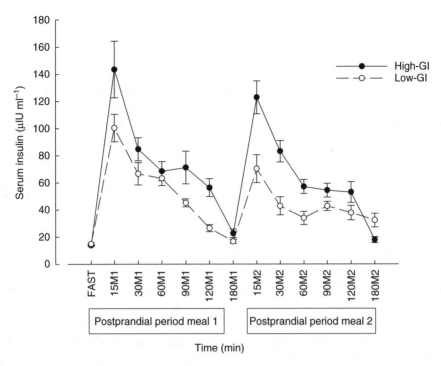

Figure 1.7 Serum insulin concentrations of seven male recreational runners following the ingestion of a high-GI (●) and a low-GI (○) breakfast and a high-GI and low-GI lunch (all meals provided 2g CHO kg^{-1} body mass; GI values for the high-GI and low-GI breakfasts were 77 and 44, respectively, and for the high-GI and low-GI lunches they were 73 and 38, respectively (adapted from Stevenson et al.[64]))

1.10 Fluid Intake Before Exercise

Drinking before exercise helps to delay the onset of severe dehydration, but the type of fluid taken should be chosen with care. Water empties from the stomach quickly but crosses the walls of the small intestine only slowly.

Adding sodium salts to water speeds up the transport of water into the systemic circulation because of the active transport of sodium. Adding some glucose also improves the absorption of fluid, but if the glucose solution is too concentrated then gastric emptying is delayed.[70] Commercially available carbohydrate–electrolyte solutions (sports drinks) with a concentration within the range 5–8% carbohydrate appear to be most effective at supplying both fluid and fuel. The gastric emptying rate of a solution is also influenced by the volume of fluid ingested. Other things being equal, a large volume empties more quickly from the stomach than a smaller volume.[71] One strategy for rapid rehydration is to drink about 120–150 ml of fluid every 15–20 min so that the volume in the stomach does not fall to the point where emptying rate slows down.

Drinking carbohydrate–electrolyte solutions before exercise does produce, during exercise, rapid rises in blood glucose and insulin concentrations, followed by a sharp fall in blood glucose. However, as exercise continues, blood glucose concentrations normally return to pre-exercise values. It is interesting to note that, even on the occasions when blood glucose concentrations fall to hypoglycaemic values during the early part of prolonged exercise, the subjects in these studies do not report any adverse sensations.[72] In summary, the weight of the available evidence does not support the commonly held view that drinking glucose solutions before exercise leads to a reduction in exercise capacity. Nevertheless, concentrated glucose solutions (10–25 per cent) are not recommended as a means of increasing carbohydrate stores within the hour before exercise because of the potential for causing gastrointestinal discomfort.

Carbohydrate intake during exercise

Drinking carbohydrate–electrolyte solutions immediately before and throughout exercise does not produce the same fall in blood glucose as that which occurs when the same solution is ingested within the hour before exercise. One of the reasons for this different response is the failure of insulin to increase in response to the elevated blood glucose concentration during exercise because the release of insulin from the pancreas is suppressed by the exercise-induced rise in plasma catecholamines.[73] Drinking carbohydrate–electrolyte solutions throughout prolonged exercise provides fluid and fuel, and so helps to delay the onset of severe dehydration and glycogen depletion.[74–76]

The improvement in endurance capacity following the ingestion of a carbohydrate–electrolyte solution throughout exercise has been attributed to an increased rate of carbohydrate oxidation while maintaining normal blood glucose concentrations.[77] More recent studies, using running rather than cycling, show that ingesting glucose–electrolyte solutions exerts a glycogen-sparing effect and this may be the underlying reason for the improvements in endurance running capacity (for review see Tsintzas et al.[78]) This glycogen sparing may not be confined to skeletal muscles but may include liver glycogen stores. Drinking carbohydrate solutions immediately before and during exercise decreases hepatic glucose production that is sustained in proportion to the amount of carbohydrate ingested.[79] The maximum rate of carbohydrate oxidation during exercise following the ingestion of carbohydrate solutions of various concentrations is approximately $1 g\ min^{-1}$.[79]

Carbohydrate intake and recovery from exercise

Rapid recovery from heavy training or competition is particularly important to sportsmen and women who have to perform every day for several days or weeks, and it is essential that they adopt a nutritional strategy which will aid rapid recovery. Central to the recovery process is the restoration of muscle and liver glycogen stores, which may have been severely depleted during exercise.

Immediately after exercise, muscle begins resynthesizing the glycogen used up during exercise. The maximum rate of glycogen resynthesis occurs during the first few hours of recovery, and so ingesting carbohydrate during this period capitalizes on this process. Ivy suggested that, in order to maximize the glycogen resynthesis rate, the optimum post-exercise carbohydrate intake should be about 1 g kg^{-1} body mass.[80] The practical prescription is 50 g of carbohydrate immediately after exercise and the same amount every 2 h up to the next meal.[81] Depleted muscle glycogen stores can be repleted in 24 h when a carbohydrate-rich diet is eaten during the recovery period.[82,83] This recovery diet should consist of 8–10 g carbohydrate kg^{-1} body mass, and should contain high-glycaemic-index carbohydrates during at least the early part of recovery.

The key question, however, is whether or not performance capacity is restored along with muscle glycogen stores following high-carbohydrate refeeding, and several studies have attempted to address this question. The results suggest that, as long as carbohydrate intake is increased from about 6 g kg^{-1} body mass per day to 9 g kg^{-1}, then endurance capacity is restored along with muscle glycogen stores.[84]

Even when the recovery period is only a few hours, and so too short to significantly increase muscle glycogen stores, there are benefits to be gained from drinking carbohydrate–electrolyte solutions. For example, Fallowfield and colleagues reported that, when runners drank a commercially available sports drink which provided the equivalent of 1 g kg^{-1} body mass of carbohydrate immediately after prolonged exercise, and again after 2 h, they were able to run for about 60 min, whereas after drinking a sweet placebo they were able to run for only 40 min.[85] Furthermore, drinking a carbohydrate–electrolyte solution is a more effective rehydrating strategy than drinking water during recovery from exercise.[86]

The type of carbohydrate consumed during the recovery period influences the rate of glycogen resynthesis.[87,88] Burke and colleagues reported that a recovery diet that contained high-GI carbohydrates resulted in a larger muscle glycogen store 24 h after prolonged exercise than after consuming a low-GI carbohydrate diet.[88] Although this study showed greater glycogen accumulation following the ingestion of a high-GI carbohydrate recovery diet, it did not include an assessment of the recovery of exercise capacity. Therefore, Stevenson and colleagues examined the influence of high- and low-GI carbohydrate recovery diets on subsequent exercise capacity.[89] Recreational runners completed 90 min of treadmill running at 70 per cent VO$_{2max}$ and were then assigned a recovery diet containing either high- or low-GI carbohydrates. Twenty-two hours later, after an overnight fast, they again ran on the treadmill, but on this occasion they continued to the point of fatigue. On the low-GI carbohydrate recovery diet they ran for 109 min and after the high-GI carbohydrate diet they ran for only 97 min. All the subjects reported that they rarely felt hungry on the low-GI carbohydrate diet whereas on the high-GI recovery diet there were times when they felt that they could have eaten more of the energy-matched meals.

There is evidence to suggest that adding some protein to the carbohydrate solution increases the rate of post-exercise glycogen synthesis to a greater extent than can be achieved with a carbohydrate solution alone.[90] The addition of protein increases the concentration of plasma insulin beyond that which is achieved with carbohydrate solutions alone after exercise. The presence of insulin stimulates the GLUT 4 transport proteins to remain active for longer than would be the case without an increased presence of this hormone.[15] As a result there is a continued increased rate of glucose transport of glucose across the muscle cell membrane that enhances glycogen resynthesis. However, when larger amounts of carbohydrate (>1.2 g/ kg body mass) are ingested during the recovery period, then the addition of protein appears not to provide an additional increase in the rate of glycogen resynthesis.[91]

As mentioned earlier, glucose uptake by muscle is greater after exercise than before exercise. Exercise changes the characteristics of the muscle membrane so that glucose permeability is improved and muscles have increased insulin sensitivity. The two effects appear to be additive. In addition, glycogen synthase, the enzyme complex responsible for glycogen synthesis, is in its most active form immediately after exercise. There is an inverse relationship between muscle glycogen concentration and the amount of glycogen synthase in the active form,[91] and athletes with the lowest post-exercise muscle glycogen concentrations show the greatest increase over the next 24 h.[92]

More recent studies have shown that the increase in post-exercise glucose uptake is associated with an increase in the glucose transporter protein, GLUT 4, after exercise.[93] Training brings about an increase in the amount of GLUT 4 (by about 50 per cent) with a parallel increase in the activity of hexokinase. It is probable that the rapid uptake of glucose is mainly the result of the presence of an increased amount of glucose transporter proteins.[94] These may enable an increase in the rate of glycogen resynthesis to occur, even when glycogen synthase levels have fallen to pre-exercise values.

1.11   Summary

This chapter has provided an overview of the relevant physiological responses to exercise and training. In addition it has included the nutritional strategies that help delay the onset of fatigue, namely how best to optimize the pre-exercise carbohydrate stores and the use of muscle glycogen during prolonged exercise. Taking regular exercise has huge health benefits that include the control of blood glucose in particular and an increase in functional capacity in general. For those people who are preparing for a prolonged period of heavy exercise, whether it is training or competition, then the recommendation is clear; they should taper their training during the week before the event and increase the carbohydrate content of their diet such that over the 48 h before the event they consume the equivalent of 8–10 g of carbohydrate kg^{-1} body weight a day. This prescription is the same for those people who have only 24 h in which to recover between training sessions or competitions. When recovery is limited to 24 h, then the high-GI carbohydrates are recommended immediately after exercise, followed by low-GI carbohydrates for the remainder of the recovery period. However, during recovery periods lasting several days or more, the type of carbohydrate consumed is not as important as during shorter recovery periods. One of the limitations to exercise, especially in the heat, is dehydration. Drinking well-formulated carbohydrate–electrolyte solutions (some sports drinks) containing no more than about 6–8 per cent carbohydrate is a good strategy to decrease the rate of dehydration during exercise and provides carbohydrate as extra fuel. The recommended amounts are of the order of 120–150 ml solution every 15–20 min. This practice improves endurance running capacity, probably by contributing to the carbohydrate metabolism in working muscles. However during exercise in very hot climates, the sports drinks should contain only about 2–4 per cent carbohydrate because under these conditions fluid is more important than fuel. After exercise rehydration is more rapid when carbohydrate–electrolyte solutions are consumed because when drinking water thirst is quenched before rehydration is achieved. One further point to note for those who have only a limited time in which to rehydrate after exercise is that they need to drink the equivalent of 150 per cent of the sweat lost. This translates into drinking in litres the equivalent of 150 per cent the body mass loss in kilograms.

The question about the optimum pre-exercise meal is still unanswered but there is growing evidence to suggest that it should contain low-GI carbohydrates. The advantages of a pre-exercise meal which contains predominantly low-GI carbohydrates is that it causes only minor perturbations of plasma glucose and insulin, and so favours a greater rate of fat metabolism. A greater rate of fat oxidation spares the limited muscle glycogen stores and so helps delay the onset of fatigue. Furthermore, when such meals are consumed 3–4 h before exercise they provide a sense of satiety for most of the postprandial period.

In conclusion, next to being born with the appropriate genes and undertaking the right training, a high-carbohydrate diet is one of the essential elements in the formula for success in sport and exercise. The nature of the carbohydrate may also play a significant part in preventing the onset of metabolic fatigue.

Acknowledgements

The author gratefully acknowledges the contributions of Dr Shiou-Liang Wee, Dr Ching-Lin Wu and Dr Emma Stevenson on their work on the GI diet and exercise.

References

1. Vitug A, Schneider S, Ruderman N. Exercise and type I diabetes mellitus. In: Pandolf K (ed.) *Exercise and Sports Sciences Reviews.* New York: Macmillan, 1988, pp. 285–304.
2. Wallberg-Henriksson H. Exercise and diabetes mellitus. In: Holloszy J (ed.), *Exercise and Sport Sciences Reviews.* Baltimore, MD: Williams & Wilkins, 1992, pp. 339–368.
3. Ramsbottom R, Brewer B, Williams C. A progressive shuttle run test to estimate maximal oxygen uptake. *Br. J. Sports Med.* 1988; **22**: 141–144.
4. Skinner J, Jaskolski A, Jaskolska A, Krasnoff J, Gagnon J, Leon A, Rao DC, Wilmore JH, Bouchard C. Age, sex, race, initial fitness and response to training: the Heritage Family Study. *J. Appl. Physiol.* 2001; **90**: 1770–1776.
5. Ramsbottom R, Nute MGL, Williams C. Determinants of five kilometre running performance in active men and women. *Br. J. Sports Med.* 1987; **21**: 9–13.
6. Costill DL, Thomason H, Roberts E. Fractional utilization of aerobic capacity during distance running. *Med. Sci. Sport* 1973; **5**: 248–252.
7. Ekblom B. Effect of physical training on oxygen transport system in man. *Acta Physiol. Scand.* 1968 (suppl. 328).
8. Hawkins S, Wisewell R. Rate and mechanisms of maximum oxygen consumption decline with aging. *Sports Med.* 2003; **33**: 877–888.
9. Brotherhood J, Brozovic B, Pugh L. Haematological status of middle and long distance runners. *Clin. Sci. Mol. Med.* 1975; **48**: 139–145.
10. Eichner E. The anemias of athletes. *Phys. Sports Med.* 1986; **14**: 123–130.
11. Ingjer F. Effects of endurance training on muscle fibre ATPase activity, capillary supply and mitochondrial content in man. *J. Physiol.* 1979; **294**: 419–432.
12. Clausen JP. Effect of physical training on cardiovascular adjustments to exercise in man. *Physiol. Rev.* 1977; **57**: 779–815.
13. Delp MD. Differential effects of training on the control of skeletal muscle perfusion. *Med. Sci. Sports Exerc.* 1998; **30**: 361–374.
14. Hickner R, Fisher J, Hansen P, Racette S, Mier C, Turner M, Holloszy JO. Muscle glycogen accumulation after endurance exercise in trained and untrained individuals. *J. Appl. Physiol.* 1997; **83**: 897–903.
15. Ivy JL, Kuo C-H. Regulation of GLUT 4 protein and glycogen synthase during muscle glycogen synthesis after exercise. *Acta Physiol. Scand.* 1998; **162**: 293–304.
16. Hyo J, Lee J, Kim J. Effect of exercise training on muscle glucose transport 4 protein and intramuscular lipid content in elderly men with impaired glucose tolerance. *Eur. J. Appl. Physiol.* 2004; **93**: 353–358.
17. McCoy M, Proietto J, Hargreaves M. Effect of detraining on GLUT 4 protein in human skeletal muscle. *J. Appl. Physiol.* 1994; **77**: 1532–1536.
18. ACSM. Exercise and type 2 diabetes. *Med. Sci. Sports Exerc.* 2000; **32**: 1345–1360.
19. Costill DL, Daniels J, Evans W, Fink W, Krehenbuhl G, Saltin B. Skeletal muscle enzymes and fiber composition in male and female track athletes. *J. Appl. Physiol.* 1976; **40**: 149–154.
20. Gollnick P, Armstrong R, Sembrowich W, Shepherd R, Saltin B. Glycogen depletion pattern in human skeletal muscle fibers after heavy exercise. *J. Appl. Physiol.* 1973; **34**: 615–618.
21. Vollestad N, Vaage O, Hermansen L. Muscle glycogen depletion patterns in type I and subgroups of type II fibres during prolonged severe exercise in man. *Acta Physiol. Scand.* 1984; **122**: 433–441.
22. Astrand P-O, Rodahl K, Dahl H, Stromme S. *Textbook of Work Physiology,* 4th edn. Champain, IL: Human Kinetics, 2003.

23. Davis JA. Anaerobic threshold: review of the concept and direction for future research. *Med. Sci. Sports Exerc.* 1985; **17**: 15–18.

24. Wasserman K, MacIlroy MB. Detecting the threshold of anaerobic metabolism in cardiac patients during exercise. *Am. J. Cardiol.* 1964; **14**: 844–852.

25. Wasserman K, Whipp B, Koyal SN, Beaver W. Anaerobic threshold and respiratory gas exchange during exercise. *J. Appl. Physiol.* 1973; **35**: 236–243.

26. Ivy JL, Withers RT, Van Handel PJ, Elger DH, Costill DL. Muscle respiratory capacity and fiber type as determinants of the lactate threshold. *J. Appl. Physiol.* 1980; **48**: 523–527.

27. Yoshida T, Nagata A, Muro M, Takuechi N, Suda Y. The validity of anaerobic threshold determination by a Douglas Bag method compared with arterial blood lactate concentration. *Eur. J. Appl. Physiol.* 1981; **46**: 423–430.

28. Brooks G. Anaerobic threshold: review of the concept and directions for future research. *Med. Sci. Sports Exerc.* 1985; **17**: 22–31.

29. Connett RJ, Honig CR, Gayeski TEJ, Brooks GA. Defining hypoxia: a systems view of VO_2, glycolysis, energetics and intracellular pO_2. *J. Appl. Physiol.* 1990; **68**: 833–842.

30. Sjodin B, Jacobs I, Svendenhag J. Changes in onset of blood lactate accumulation (OBLA) and muscle enzymes after training at OBLA. *Eur. J. Appl. Physiol.* 1982; **49**: 45–57.

31. Kindermann W, Simon G, Keul J. The significance of the aerobic-anaerobic transition for the determination of work load intensities during endurance training. *Eur. J. Appl. Physiol.* 1979; **42**: 25–34.

32. Ramsbottom R, Williams C, Boobis L, Freeman W. Aerobic fitness and running performance of male and female recreational runners. *J. Sports Sci.* 1989; **7**: 9–20.

33. Coyle EF, Coggan AR, Hopper MK, Walters TJ. Determinants of endurance in well-trained cyclists. *J. Appl. Physiol.* 1988; **64**: 2622–2630.

34. Williams C, Brewer J, Patton A. The metabolic challenge of the marathon. *Br. J. Sports Med.* 1984; **18**: 245–252.

35. Billatt V, Sirvent P, Py G, Koralsztein J, Mercier J. The concept of maximal lactate steady-state. *Sports Med.* 2003; **33**: 407–426.

36. Boobis LH. Metabolic aspects of fatigue during sprinting. In: Macleod D, Maughan R, Nimmo M, Reilly T, Williams C (eds), *Exercise, Benefits, Limitations and Adaptations.* London: Spon, 1987, pp. 116–140.

37. Helge J, Richter E, Kiens B. Interaction of training and diet on metabolism and endurance during exercise in man. *J. Physiol.* 1996; **492**: 293–306.

38. Burke L, Angus D, Cox G, Cummings N, Fabbraio M, Gawthorn K Hawley JA, Mirchan M, Martin DT, Hargreaves M. Effect of fat adaptation and carbohydrate restoration on metabolism and performance during prolonged cycling. *J. Appl. Physiol.* 2000; **89**: 2413–2421.

39. Burke L, Hawley J, Angus D, Cox G, Clark S, Cummings N, Desbrow B, Hargreaves M. Adaptations to short-term high-fat diet persist during exercise despite high carbohydrate availability. *Med. Sci. Sport Exerc.* 2002; **34**: 83–91.

40. Carey A, Staudacher H, Cummings N, Steptoe N, Nikolopoulos V, Burke E *et al.* Effects of fat adaptation and carbohydrate restoration on prolonged endurance exercise. *J. Appl. Physiol.* 2001; **91**: 115–122.

41. Stephen A, Sieber G, Gerster Y, Morgan R. Intake of carbohydrate and its components-international comparison: trends over time, and effects of changing to a low fat diet. *Am. J. Clin. Nutr.* 1995; **62**: 851S–867S.

42. Janssen G, Graef C, Saris W. Food intake and body composition in novice athletes during a training period to run a marathon. *Int. J. Sports Med.* 1989; **10**(supplement1): S17–S21.

43. Williams C. Carbohydrate needs of elite athletes. In: Simopoulos A, Pavlou K (eds), *Nutrition and Fitness of Athletes.* New York: Karger, 1993, pp. 34–60.

44. Devlin J, Williams C. Foods, nutrition and sports performance; a final consensus statement. *J. Sports Sci.* 1991; **9** (Suppl): iii.

45. Ekblom B, Williams C. Foods, nutrition and soccer performance: final consensus statement. *J. Sports Sci.* 1994; 12(special issue):S3.

46. Maughan R, Horton E. Current issues in nutrition in athletics. *J. Sports Sci.* 1995; **13S**: 1S–90S.

47. Sherman W, Costill D, Fink W, Miller J. Effect of exercise-diet manipulation on muscle glycogen and its subsequent utilization during performance. *Int. J. Sports Med.* 1981; **2**: 114–118.

48. Bergstrom J, Hermansen L, Hultman E, Saltin B. Diet, muscle glycogen and physical performance. *Acta Physiol. Scand.* 1967; **71**: 140–150.

49. Conlee R. Muscle glycogen and exercise endurance: a twenty year prospective. In: Pandolf K (ed.), *Exercise and Sports Science Reviews*. London: Collier Macmillan; 1987, pp. 1–28.

50. Goforth HW, Hodgdon JA, Hilderbrand RL. A double blind study of the effects of carbohydrate loading upon endurance performance. *Med. Sci. Sport Exerc.* 1980;**12**: 108A.

51. Brewer J, Williams C, Patton A. The influence of high carbohydrate diets on endurance running performance. *Eur. J. Appl. Physiol.* 1988; **57**: 698–706.

52. Karlsson J, Saltin B. Diet, muscle glycogen and endurance performance. *J. Appl. Physiol.* 1971; **31**: 203–206.

53. Sherman W, Costill D, Fink W, Miller J. Effect of exercise-diet manipulation on muscle glycogen and its subsequent utilization during performance. *Int. J. Sports Med.* 1981; **2**: 114–118.

54. Maughan RJ, Williams C, Campbell DM, Hepburn D. Fat and carbohydrate metabolism during low intensity exercise: effects of the availability of muscle glycogen. *Eur. J. Appl. Physiol.* 1978; **39**: 7–16.

55. Saltin B. Metabolic fundamentals of exercise. *Med. Sci. Sports Exerc.* 1973; **15**: 366–369.

56. Tarnopolsky LJ, MacDougall JD, Atkinson SA, Tarnopolsky MA, Sutton JR. Gender differences in substrate for endurance exercise. *J. Appl. Physiol.* 1990; **68**: 302–307.

57. Tarnopolsky M. Nutritional implications of gender differences in energy metabolism. In: Driskell J, Wolinsky I (eds), *Energy-yielding Macronutrients and Energy Metabolism in Sports Nutrition*. London: CRC Press, 2000, pp. 245–262.

58. Walker L, Heigenhauser G, Hultman E, Spriet L. Dietary carbohydrate, muscle glycogen content, and endurance performance in well trained women. *J. Appl. Physiol.* 2000; **88**: 2151–2158.

59. Jenkins DJA, Thomas DM, Wolever MS, Taylor RH, Barker H, Fielden H, Baldwin JM, Bowling AC, Newman HC, Jerkins Al, Goff DV. Glycemic index of foods: a physiological basis for carbohydrate exchange. *Am. J. Clin. Nutr.* 1981; **34**: 362–366.

60. Foster-Powell K, Brand Miller J. International tables of glycemic index. *Am. J. Clin. Nutr.* 1995;**62**: 871S–893S.

61. Rankin W. Glycemic Index and exercise metabolism. *Sports Sci. Exch.* 1997; **10**: 1–6.

62. Thomas D, Brotherhood J, Brand J. Carbohydrate feeding before exercise: effect of glycemic index. *Int. J. Sports Med.* 1991; **12**: 180–186.

63. Wee S, Williams C, Tsintzas K, Boobis L. Effect of high and low glycaemic index pre-exercise meals on muscle glycogen and exercise metabolism. In: Parisi P, Pigozzi F, Prinzi G (eds), *4th Annual Congress of the European College of Sports Sciences*. Rome: University Institute of Motor Sciences, 1999, p. 44.

64. Stevenson E, Williams C, Nute M. The influence of glycaemic index of breakfast and lunch on substrate utilisation during postprandial periods and subsequent exercise. *Br. J. Nutr.* 2005; **93**: 885–893.

65. Wee S-L, Williams C, Gray S, Horabin J. Influence of high and low glycemic index meals on endurance running capacity. *Med. Sci. Sport. Exerc.* 1999; **31**: 393–399.

66. Wu C-L, Nicholas C, Williams C, Took A, Hardy L. The influence of high-carbohydrate meals with different glycaemic indices on substrate utilisation during subsequent exercise. *Br. J. Nutr.* 2003; **90**: 1049–1056.

67. Kirwan J, O'Gorman D, Evans W. A moderate glycemic meal before endurance exercise can enhance performance. *J. Appl. Physiol.* 1998; **84**: 53–59.

68. Wu C-L, Williams C. Influence of pre-exercise high carbohydrate breakfast with different glycaemic indices on running endurance capacity and substrate utilisation in men. *In. J. Sport Nutr. Exerc. Metab.* 2005 (in press).

69. Febbraio M, Stewart K. CHO feeding before prolonged exercise: effect of glycemic index on muscle glycogenolysis and exercise performance. *J. Appl. Physiol.* 1996; **82**: 1115–1120.

70. Vist G, Maughan R. Gastric emptying of ingested solutions in man: effect of beverage glucose concentration. *Med. Sci. Sports Exerc.* 1994; **26**: 1269–1273.

71. Noakes TD, Rehrer NJ, Maughan RJ. The importance of volume in regulating gastric emptying. *Med. Sci. Sports Exerc.* 1991; **23**: 307–313.

72. Chryssanthopoulos C, Hennessy L, Williams C. The Influence of pre-exercise glucose ingestion on endurance running capacity. *Br. J. Sports Med.* 1994; **28**: 105–109.

73. Porte D, Williamson R. Inhibition of insulin release by norepinephrine in man. *Science* 1966; **152**: 1248–1250.

74. Murray R. Fluid needs in hot and cold environments. *Int. J. Sport Nutr.* 1995;**5**: S62–S73.

75. Tsintzas O, Williams C, Singh R, Wilson W, Burrin J. Influence of carbohydrate-electrolyte drinks on marathon running performance. *Eur. J. Appl. Physiol.* 1995; **70**: 154–160.

76. Tsintzas O-K, Williams C, Boobis L, Greenhaff P. Carbohydrate ingestion and glycogen utilization in different muscle fibre types in man. *J. Physiol.* 1995; **489**: 243–250.

77. Coyle EF, Coggan AR, Hemmert MK, Ivy JL. Muscle glycogen utilization during prolonged strenuous exercise when fed carbohydrate. *J. Appl. Physiol.* 1986; **61**: 165–172.

78. Tsintzas K, Williams C. Human muscle glycogen metabolism during exercise: effect of carbohydrate supplementation. *Sports Med.* 1998; **25**: 7–23.

79. Jeukendrup A, Jentjens R. Oxidation of carbohydrate feedings during prolonged exercise: current thoughts, guidelines and directions for future directions. *Sports Med* 2000; **29**: 407–424.

80. Ivy JL. Muscle glycogen synthesis before and after exercise. *Sports Med.* 1991; **11**: 6–19.

81. Coyle E. Timing and method of increased carbohydrate intake to cope with heavy training, competition and recovery. *J. Sports Sci.* 1991; **19**(special issue): S29–S52.

82. Bergstrom J, Hultman E. Muscle glycogen synthesis after exercise: an enhancing factor localized to the muscle cell in man. *Nature* 1966; **20**: 309–310.

83. Keizer H, Kuipers H, van Kranenburg G. Influence of liquid and solid meals on muscle glycogen resynthesis, plasma fuel hormone reponses, and maximal physical working capacity. *Int. J. Sports Med.* 1987; **8**: 99–104.

84. Fallowfield J, Williams C. Carbohydrate intake and recovery from prolonged exercise. *Int. J. Sport Nutr.* 1993; **3**: 150–164.

85. Fallowfield J, Williams C, Singh R. The influence of ingesting a carbohydrate–electrolyte solution during 4 hours recovery from prolonged running on endurance capacity. *Int. J. Sport Nutr.* 1995; **5**: 285–299.

86. Gonzalez-Alonso J, Heaps CL, Coyle EF. Rehydration after exercise with common beverages and water. *Int. J. Sports Med.* 1992; **13**: 399–406.

87. Keins B. Translating nutrition into diet: diet for training and competition. In: Macleod D, Maughan R, Williams C, Madeley C, Sharp J, Nutton R (eds), *Intermittent High Intensity*

Exercise: Preparation, Stresses and Damage Limitation. London: Spon, 1993, pp. 175–182.

88. Burke L, Collier G, Hargreaves M. Muscle glycogen storage after prolonged exercise: effect of the glycaemic index of carbohydrate feedings. *J. Appl. Physiol.* 1993; **75**: 1019–1023.

89. Stevenson E, Williams C, McCombe G, Oram, C. Improved recovery from prolonged exercise following the consumption of low glycaemic index carbohydrate meals. *Int. J. Sport Nutr. Exerc. Metab.* 2005; **15**: 333–349.

90. Zawadzki K, Yaspelkis III B, Ivy J. Carbohydrate-protein complex increases the rate of muscle glycogen storage after exercise. *J. Appl. Physiol.* 1992; **72**: 1854–1859.

91. Jentjens R, Jeukendrupt A. Determinants of post-exercise glycogen resynthesis during short term recovery. *Sports Med.* 2003; **33**: 117–144.

92. Jacobs I, Westlin N, Karlsson J, Rasmusson M, Houghton B. Muscle glycogen and diet in elite soccer players. *Eur. J. Appl. Physiol.* 1982; **48**: 297–302.

93. McCoy M, Proietto J, Hargreaves M. Skeletal muscle Glut 4 and post-exercise muscle glycogen storage in humans. *J. Appl. Physiol.* 1996; **80**: 411–415.

94. Nakatani A, Han D-H, Hansen P, Nolte L, Host H, Hickner R, Holloszy JO. Effect of endurance exercise training on muscle glycogen supercompensation in rats. *J. Appl. Physiol.* 1997; **82**: 711–715.

2

Exercise in Type 1 Diabetes

Jean-Jacques Grimm

2.1 Introduction

Regular exercise in people with diabetes does not necessarily lead to improved control. Indeed, the metabolic disturbances associated with sustained exercise may lead to worsening control unless great care is taken to adjust carbohydrate intake and the insulin dosage. Type 1 diabetes frequently affects children, adolescents and young adults in whom health improvement does not feature highly among the reasons for exercising. The desire to play, or to become a member of a team, is often more important, and is driven by social reasons and the need not to appear 'different' from the peer group. The aim of the medical team is to allow the diabetic child or adult to participate in the sport of his or her choice and to avoid any form of discrimination during school sports or when playing on a team.

This chapter deals with the way a person with type 1 diabetes could manage their condition independently and safely during various kinds of sports and recreation.

Recent literature[1,2] acknowledges that 'all levels of exercise, including leisure activities, recreational sports, and competitive professional activities (www.steveredgrave.com/), can be performed by people with type 1 diabetes'. It must be stressed, however, that high-intensity endurance exercise (e.g. marathon, triathlon, cross-country skiing) is not required to achieve maximal health benefits from exercise.[3] Regular, moderate-intensity exercise[1,4] has the best risk–benefit ratio.

The advantages of exercise in type 1 diabetes relate more to its protective cardiovascular effects than to improved glycaemic control. Exercise is not a tool for improving blood glucose control in type 1 diabetes. However, the diabetes education team needs to be knowledgeable about all treatment adjustments

Exercise and Sport in Diabetes, 2nd Edition   Edited by Dinesh Nagi
© 2005 John Wiley & Sons, Ltd.

required to enable their patients to exercise safely and with maximum health benefits; regular exercise may improve insulin sensitivity in the overweight type 1 diabetic person and therefore render blood glucose control easier.

2.2   Exercise Physiology

As well as an increase in oxygen availability, exercise requires rapid mobilization and redistribution of metabolic fuels to ensure adequate energy supply for the working muscles (see Chapter 1). This necessitates a cascade of neural, cardio-vascular and hormonal adjustments.

Fuels metabolized by skeletal muscle

Skeletal muscle metabolizes mainly glucose, free fatty acids (FFA) and triglycer-ides. Ketones do not participate in the oxidative metabolism of the active muscles in the healthy human.[5] Amino acids derived from catabolism within the muscle can be used as an energy source by muscles during very long and very intense effort. Nevertheless, amino acids never contribute more than 10 per cent of the total energy expenditure.[6]

Sources and proportions of fuels used during exercise

During the first 20–30 min of effort, muscle glycogen is the main source of energy.[7] Later, blood-borne glucose derived from hepatic glycogenolysis, gluco-neogenesis and intestinal absorption is metabolized, followed by muscle triglycer-ides and circulating FFA derived from adipose tissue (Figure 2.1).

At rest almost no blood glucose enters the muscle cell. During the first 10 min of exercise, blood glucose represents 10–15 per cent of oxidative metabolism, and after 90 min it can increase to 40 per cent of the total fuel utilization.[9] After 4 h of exercise, blood glucose provides approximately one-third and FFA two-thirds of the oxidative fuels.[10] After 8 h of moderate exercise, FFAs are responsible for 80–85 per cent of the oxidative fuel, the rest being derived from glucose with a small contribution from branched-chain amino acids.[11]

Regulation of fuel delivery during exercise

During exercise of moderate intensity, insulin and glucagons are the main regulators of hepatic glucose production. A low level of plasma insulin is required

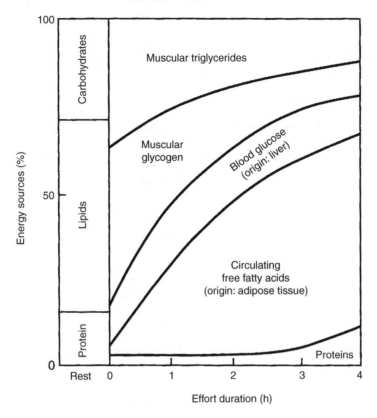

Figure 2.1 Regulation of energy sources during mild exercise of long duration. Experimental situation without glucose ingestion[8]

to allow hepatic glycogenolysis, and an increase in glucagon concentration is necessary for both glycogenolysis and gluconeogenesis.[12] The glucagon–insulin ratio correlates better with hepatic glucose production than insulin or glucagon levels alone.[13] It seems that a decrease in insulin level enhances hepatic sensitivity to the action of glucagon. Without the presence of glucagon, however, the decrease in insulin concentration alone does not stimulate hepatic glycogenolysis.[14]

Adrenaline stimulates hepatic glucose production during intense effort of long duration by facilitating mobilization of the precursors of gluconeogenesis. Catecholamines are also responsible for extra glucose production during very intense exercises of short duration.[15,16]

Lypolysis is stimulated by increased catecholamine levels, which also suppress insulin secretion. Increased α-adrenergic stimulation from noradrenaline released from sympathetic nerves seems to be the most prominent stimulus to lipolysis,[17] together with increased sensitivity of the adipocytes to catecholamines.[18]

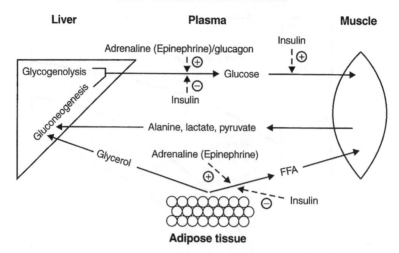

Figure 2.2 Main energy fluxes during exercise, and their regulation in blood glucose homeostasis. In the non-diabetic exercising subject, the plasma insulin level decreases, whereas the adrenaline and glucagon levels increase. Adapted from Zinman[19] by permission of Lilly Research Laboratories

Consequences of diabetes on the metabolic reponse to exercise

The problems relating to blood glucose control in physically active insulin-treated people can be explained by imbalances between the plasma insulin level and the available plasma glucose. Very often the plasma insulin, derived from injected insulin, is too high during exercise compared with the insulin level of a non-diabetic person in the same situation. At the same time, the carbohydrate supply is often too low because hepatic glycogenolysis is blocked by high insulin levels (Figure 2.2).

2.3   Insulin Absorption

The importance of changing the injection site when doing sports or being physically active continues to be actively debated. Various factors speed the rate of insulin absorption, including increased blood flow to the injection site due to exercise, increased ambient temperature[21,22] or local massage.[23] There is considerable intra-individual variation in insulin absorption rate (up to 15 per cent difference for the same site from day to day[24]), and it has been shown that insulin (NPH, soluble) absorption from sites in the abdomen is significantly more rapid than that from sites in the thigh. This difference is much smaller with the short-acting insulin analogues and does not have clinical relevance.[24] In the 1970s, experimental data[25] showed that muscular activity speeds insulin absorption from an exercising limb. This was considered at least part of the explanation for the increased insulin action during exercise. Many considered that injecting the insulin in a non-exercising area would help to prevent hypoglycaemic attacks during and after exercise, but Kemmer et al.[26] showed that this strategy did not prevent effort-related hypoglycaemia. Because of the difference between various injection sites, using a different site on an on–off basis specifically for athletic activity is not recommended – this would simply add another variable. Because absorption rates vary from site to site, it is sensible to restrict short-acting insulin injections to one site. If the abdomen is used routinely, this obviates worries about varying insulin absorption rates from an exercising limb. If the basal insulin (slow acting) is injected into the thigh, we suggest not changing the injection site, but eventually decreasing the dosage, as described later in this chapter.

Risk of involuntary intramuscular injection

Intramuscular injection of insulin is a cause of hypoglycaemia[27] independent of exercise. It is clear that this risk is increased if the injection is followed by exercise. The physically active diabetic person must be informed of the need to avoid intramuscular injections and to take particular care with the injection technique.

Short needles (8.0 mm) have been marketed with the claim that they avoid the risk of intramuscular injection and obviate the need to pinch the skin. Unfortunately, it was proposed at the same time to inject without folding the skin. However, it seems that even with 8.0 mm needles some insulin injections can be intramuscular when injected without a skin-fold in lean persons. Furthermore, short needles expose the patient to the risk of intradermal injections or insulin leaks when the technique is not perfect. Consequently, we suggest routinely using a skin-fold when injecting insulin, whatever the length of the needle used (5.0, 8.0, 10.0 or 12.7 mm).

Recommendations for exercise and insulin injections

- Inject the insulin into the usual location.

- Take special care with the injection to make sure it is not intramuscular.

- Learn to adapt (decrease) the insulin dose, depending on the type, duration and timing of exercise.

- Use frequent blood glucose measurements, especially during unfamiliar activities.

2.4 Hypoglycaemia

The risk of hypoglycaemia during exercise in the insulin-dependent diabetic person was expertly described, a few years after the discovery of insulin, by the British physician R.D. Lawrence.[28] In contrast to the non-diabetic subject, where the insulin level falls shortly after exercise commences, the insulin level in the person with diabetes is governed mainly by the amount and timing of the last injection. It follows that he or she must anticipate strenuous activities and make appropriate reductions in the insulin dose. If this is not done, the only option is to take extra carbohydrate to try to compensate for excess circulating insulin.

The fear of hypoglycaemic comas has often been the cause of discrimination against children with diabetes, leading to their exclusion from gymnastics or summer camps. Some children with diabetes decide spontaneously not to participate in group or team activities, for fear of upsetting their team-mates because of the need for regular blood glucose checks and the necessity to eat snacks at precise times, or because a hypoglycaemic episode might upset the team performance.

Hypoglycaemia may happen during exercise, but also or up to 12–14 h or even longer after the end of the effort.[29,30] Late-onset hypoglycaemia is explained both by the body's need to replenish glycogen stores and by a sustained increase of the tissue sensitivity to insulin. When the exercise sessions continue for several days, insulin needs usually decrease progressively from day to day.

Repeated episodes of hypoglycaemia lead to an unfortunate vicious circle whereby there is decreased hypoglycaemic awareness, leading to the risk of more hypoglycaemia.[29] Furthermore, physical activity makes the recognition of hypoglycaemia difficult because sweating and tachycardia due to physical effort can mask similar signs warning of impending hypoglycaemia.

When hypoglycaemia happens during exercise despite all efforts to avoid it, it is often extremely difficult to treat. Very often the activity has to be temporarily suspended, and the amount of carbohydrate required to correct the blood glucose may be unusually high, often 30–40 g or more. Exercise-onset hypoglycaemia tends to be recurrent and more carbohydrate may be needed within half an hour (preferably after a repeat blood glucose test).

2.5 Hyperglycaemia

Exercise can cause a rise in blood glucose in two situations: (1) when an individual is insulin-deficient and metabolically unstable; (2) with extremely intense exercise in individuals who have well controlled diabetes.

Pre-exercise high blood glucose and ketones

This situation is the consequence of a severe deficit in circulating insulin, leading to an increase in hepatic glucose production, a decrease in glucose disposal by muscle, and the production of ketones. Furthermore, exercise stimulates the secretion of counter-regulatory hormones (glucagon, catecholamines, growth hormone and cortisol), all of which contribute to hyperglycaemia and metabolic deterioration.[30]

Hyperglycaemia (>14.0 mmol l^{-1}) with ketonuria is an absolute contraindication to exercise. The metabolic imbalance must be corrected by short-acting insulin injections and the activity must not be resumed until the blood glucose level starts to decrease and urine ketones disappear.

High blood glucose without ketones

That situation may be the consequence of a mild and relative insulin deficiency. It can be the result of an excess of carbohydrate at the last meal or snack or the consequence of stress. Exercise is allowed but with caution. Good hydration must be stressed (drink before, during and after exercise). A blood glucose measurement is recommended after 30 min of exercise. If no decrease is observed, exercise cessation is recommended and a correction insulin injection as well.

Very intense short exercise with normal blood glucose

Very intense [>80 per cent of maximal oxygen uptake (VO_{2max})] and short-duration exercise, such as weight-lifting, can increase glycaemia. The main explanation is a large increase in catecholamine production.[16] In the original work of Mitchell et al.,[15] the duration of the effort was 10 min and the intensity 80 per cent of the VO_{2max}. Two groups of diabetics were observed, a metabolically well-controlled group (mean blood glucose 4.8 mmol l^{-1}), and a less well-controlled group (mean blood glucose 8.3 mmol l^{-1}). Two hours after exercise, the increase in blood glucose was 2.9 mmol l^{-1} in the well-controlled group and 4.2 mmol l^{-1} in the less well-controlled group.

When short bouts of intense exercise are repeated many times during a limited time span (1–2 h) such as, for example, during an ice hockey game, energy consumption is considerable, and will finally lead to a decrease in blood glucose, with a risk of hypoglycaemia.

2.6   Strategies for Treatment Adjustments

Two important principles must be taken into account in making treatment adjustments before, during and after exercise in people with type 1 diabetes:

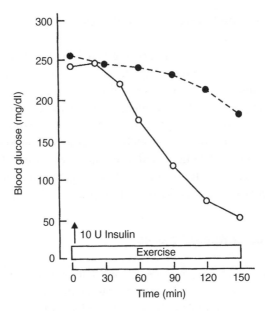

Figure 2.3 Effect of subcutaneously injected insulin at rest (•) and with muscular exercise (0)[28]

1. Exercise is always associated with extra energy consumption.

2. Exercise stimulates glucose uptake into muscle cells (increases insulin sensitivity). The same amount of insulin allows more glucose to be metabolized during an effort than at rest (Figure 2.3).

Most people with type 1 diabetes who are planning to exercise have heard about extra carbohydrates and insulin dose adjustments and are aware of the increased risk of hypoglycaemia. However, experience shows that very often they underestimate the reduction in insulin dose required. In addition to this, the need to compensate for energy expenditure with extra carbohydrate is often neglected or underestimated. This is the main cause of preventable hypoglycaemia.[33,34]

These errors become critical when, due to an excess of circulating insulin, hepatic glycogen stores cannot be mobilized and gluconeogenesis cannot occur (see Figure 2.2).

Correct preparation for exercise needs a detailed assessment of all the characteristics of the effort: duration, intensity, time from last meal and or insulin injection, time of the day and insulin activity (blood insulin level) during the exercise session. Frequent blood glucose testing is of value during the first attempts in any new activity.

- Leaving an interval of 2–3 h between the last meal/insulin injection avoids exercising during the peak insulin action where the risk of hypoglycaemia is

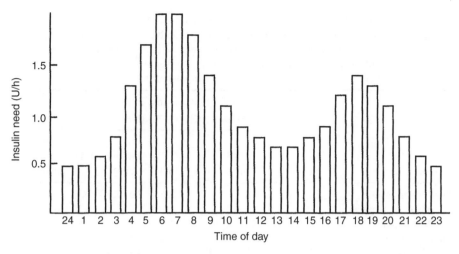

Figure 2.4 Variations of the hourly insulin needs during 24 h, independently of meals, in 198 subjects with type 1 diabetes treated by continuous subcutaneous insulin infusion pump therapy[36]

high.[35] This is valid with short-acting insulin analogues. With classical short-acting insulins it is recommended to wait 4 h or substantially decrease the meal insulin dose.

- Time of day is important, not only because insulin levels fluctuate through the day but also because the body's need for insulin is low at certain times of the day (Figure 2.4).

- Estimation of the times when insulin levels are high for every type of insulin injection is one of the important homework tasks for the would-be exerciser.[37] Table 2.1 shows 'intense' insulin activity periods for different insulin preparations and dosages. Exercising during these periods needs special attention because of the increased risk of hypoglycaemia. When exercise is supposed to take place during the 'intense' activity of a short-acting insulin, its dose must be drastically reduced and extra carbohydrates taken too.

2.7 Evaluation of the Intensity and Duration of the Effort

Intensity

Effort intensity is well correlated with heart rate (HR) in the absence of heart rhythm abnormalities or autonomic neuropathy. One way of defining the intensity of exercise is to state the actual HR as a percentage of the maximal HR. The

Table 2.1   Periods of 'intense' insulin activity of different insulin preparation and dosages. The 'period of intense insulin activity is defined as the time between the moment when insulin activity reaches two thirds and the moment when it falls below two-thirds of the peak[37] The active period of the long-acting insulin analogues glargine (Lantus[R]) and detemir (Levemir[R]) is determined differently[43] because they don't have a real peak of action

| Type of insulin | Units | Period of intense insulin (h) activity, subcutaneous injection | | | | Period of intense insulin activity (h) after subcutaneous injection |
		T 50% (h)	Start	End	Variation (end)	
Short-acting insulin analogue (Humalog,[a] Novorapid[a])	10	1.3	0.5	2.6	2.3–3.3	
Short-acting insulin (Actrapid[a])	6	2.3	1	4.6	3.5–5.8	
	12	2.7	1	5.4	4.1–6.8	
	20	3.0	1	6.0	4.5–7.5	
Basal insulins						
NPH	6	7.5	2.5	9.0	6.7–11.3	
	12	8.5	2.5	10.2	7.7–12.8	
	24	10.6	2.5	12.8	9.5–16.0	
	36	13.0	2.5	15.6	11.7–19.5	
Zinc insulins						
Monotard HM[a]	6	7.3	3.0	8.8	6.6–11.0	
	12	8.9	3.0	10.7	8.8–13.4	
	24	10.9	3.0	13.1	9.8–16.4	
	36	14.8	3.0	17.8	13.3–22.3	
Ultratard HM[a]	6	13.0	4–6	15.6	11.7–19.5	
	24	15.1	4–6	18.1	13.6–22.6	
Semi lente[a]	40	8.0	2.5	12.0	9.0–15.0	
Long-acting insulin analogues[*]						
Lantus	0.3 U/kg		1.5	22	18.3–25.7	
	0.2 U/kg		1.0	15.2		
Levemir	0.4 U/kg		1.0	21.5		

[*]Due to less scientific research data, the long acting analogues are presented in a different way compared to the other insulins. To give the U/kg a real meaning to you, multiply it by your weight in kg. The begin and the end of the insulin action are also calculated on a different basis.

maximal HR can be calculated or measured during a bicycle or treadmill stress test. Calculated (theoretical) maximal HR for all women or untrained men is 220 minus age. For trained men, it is $205 - 0.5 \times$ age.[38]

Example 1: calculation of maximal HR

- Untrained 50-year-old man; maximal HR, $220 - 50 = 170$ beats min^{-1}.

- Trained 50-year-old man. Maximal HR, $205 - 20 = 185$ beats min^{-1}.

Table 2.2 Extra carbohydrate amounts and insulin dose reductions for different sessions. The values in bold show situations where an insulin dosage reduction is required

Intensity (Percentage of maximum HR)	Duration (min)		
	Short (<20)	Medium (20–60)	Long (>60)
Low (<60)	0–10 g	10–20 g	15–30 g/h
Moderate (60–75)	10–20 g	20–60 g	20–100 g/h
High (>75)	0–30 g	30–100 g	30–100 g/h

Exercise intensity is defined according to the following formula:

- low-intensity exercise, <60 per cent of maximal HR;

- moderate-intensity exercise, 60–75 per cent of maximal HR;

- high-intensity exercise, >75 per cent of maximal HR.

Example 2: estimation of exercise intensity

- A 40-year-old woman, HR during exercise 80 beats min^{-1}; maximal HR, $220 - 40 = 180$ beats min^{-1}; HR/maximal HR $= 80/180 = 45$ per cent. This exercise is of low intensity.

Duration

Short <20 min; medium 20–60 min; long >60 min.

Characterization of the effort

Table 2.2 shows nine combinations of different durations and intensities of exercise. Every exercise session can be characterized with this chart.

2.8 Nutritional Treatment Adaptations

Without energy, there can be no exercise! The energy comes from stores located in the body or from ingested food or beverages. The diabetic person relies more than non-diabetic subjects on an adequate energy intake before, during and after exercise.

Although glucose represents only a part of the fuel metabolized during exercise, for simplification during patient education it is suggested that the energy expended must be replaced in the form of glucose, or carbohydrate equivalent, during and after exertion. People with diabetes whose insulin dosage has been adequately reduced need at least as much extra glucose during an effort as non-diabetics.[39]

Carbohydrate supplementation alone will prevent most hypoglycaemic episodes.[34] Precise counselling in carbohydrate supplementation is extremely difficult, but Table 2.2 provides a guide for the approximate amounts of additional carbohydrate required for exercises of different duration and intensity. The amounts of carbohydrate have been validated in adults doing different activities [callisthenics, walking, mountain biking (personal data)].

The proposed extra carbohydrate intakes are rough estimates, with relatively wide ranges. It is possible to increase the precision (make the range narrower) by comparing with the amounts listed in Table 2.3, which gives estimates of carbohydrate requirements for particular sports and activities and for three different body weights.[37]

Although these tables give some indication of the energy expenditure associated with different activities and provide a starting point from which to make adjustments, at the end of the day there is no substitute for experience and for trial and (hopefully not too much) error. An important point is that the plasma insulin level at the start of exercise is never known. It can, however, be roughly estimated by observation of the slope between two blood glucose measurements at 15 and 30 min before exercise. A pronounced fall would indicate that additional carbohydrate is likely to be needed.

For endurance activities (several hours), the hourly need for extra carbohydrate will often reduce for two reasons:

1. a shift towards FFA consumption rather than glucose by the active muscle;

2. a drifting away from the period of maximal insulin action (in most cases) and decreased risk of insulin excess.

The relative amount of carbohydrate of FFA oxidized during an endurance effort will depend on the patient's fitness level. Trained athletes oxidize FFA earlier and in greater amounts than untrained athletes and will spare carbohydrates in this way.

2.9 Insulin Dose Adjustment

Even the most elaborate insulin treatment scheme (subcutaneous insulin infusion pump or multiple insulin injections) cannot mimic the subtle insulin adjustments of a healthy pancreas. The most common failing of insulin therapy, compared with

Table 2.3 Grams of carbohydrate used each hour in common activities[37]

| Activity | Grams of CHO used per hour by weight | | | Approximate percentage of total calories from CHO |
	100 lb (45 kg)	150 lb (68 kg)	200 lb (90 kg)	
Baseball	25	38	50	40
Basketball:				
moderate	35	53	70	50
vigorous	59	89	118	60
Bicycling:				
6 mph	20	27	34	40
10 mph	35	48	61	50
14 mph	60	83	105	60
18 mph	95	130	165	65
20 mph	122	168	214	70
Dancing:				
moderate	17	25	33	40
vigorous	28	43	57	50
Digging	45	65	83	50
Eating	6	8	10	30
Golfing (pullcart)	23	35	46	40
Handball	59	88	117	60
Jump rope, 80 min^{-1}	73	109	145	65
Mopping	12	18	24	30
Mountain climbing	60	90	120	60
Outside painting	21	31	42	40
Raking leaves	19	28	38	30
Running:				
5 mph	45	68	90	50
8 mph	96	145	190	65
10 mph	126	189	252	70
Shovelling	31	45	57	50
Skating:				
moderate	25	34	43	40
vigorous	67	92	117	60
Skiing:				
cross-country, 5 mph	76	105	133	60
downhill	52	72	92	50
water	42	58	74	50
Soccer	45	67	89	50
Swimming:				
slow crawl	41	56	71	50
fast crawl	69	95	121	60
Tennis:				
moderate	28	41	55	40
vigorous	59	88	117	60
Volleyball:				
moderate	23	34	45	40
vigorous	59	88	117	60
Walking:				
3 mph	15	22	29	30
4.5 mph	30	45	59	45

Table 2.4   Decrease in insulin dosage for efforts of different intensities and durations

Intensity (Percentage of maximum HR)	Duration (min)		
	<20	20–60	>60
Low (<60), e.g. walking, slow swimming	— —		Prandial insulin, 5–10% = h exercise Basal insulin, 5–10% = h exercise
Moderate (60–70): e.g. hiking, cycling, jogging	—	Prandial insulin: 10–50% Basal insulin: 10–20%	Prandial insulin, 5–10% = h exercise Basal insulin, 5–10% = h exercise
High (>75): e.g. mountain biking, running, competition cycling or swimming	—	Prandial insulin: 10–50% Basal insulin: 10–20%	Prandial insulin, 5–20% = h exercise Basal insulin, 5–20% = h exercise

natural secretion, is a lack of insulin in the minutes following the start of a meal and an excess of insulin 3–4 h after the meal. These faults can partly be avoided with pump treatment or with subcutaneous injections of a very-short-acting insulin analogue (lispro, asparte) combined with a split (divided into two or three injections during the day) basal insulin administration (see Chapter 6).

As insulin regimens and formulations differ widely from patient to patient, the strategies must be personalized. For low-intensity exercise lasting up to 1 h, and for any higher intensity exercise lasting less than 20 min, it is usually not necessary to change the insulin dose (Table 2.4). If the starting blood glucose is low or falling, it is wise to eat a snack before starting. Table 2.4 considers the insulins which are active during *and* after exercise.

Pump treatment

The basic principles of treatment adaptations are similar to those applied with a multiple injection scheme.

Basal insulin

One of the main advantages of pump treatment when exercising is the possibility of setting a temporary basal rate. Practically the exercising person reduces his or her basal rate by 20–50 per cent, sometimes up to 80 per cent, from 1 h prior to the beginning of the effort until several hours after the end of the exercise. For exercise lasting half a day or more, the reduced basal rate (80 per cent of 100 per cent) can be maintained for the whole following night.

Prandial insulin

If the meal insulin activity overlaps the exercising time, that insulin has to be decreased. The global amounts of insulin dose reduction can be estimated in accordance with Table 2.4. The decrease in meal insulin dosage is usually about 20–50 per cent.

As with a multiple injection scheme, there is a choice between ingesting more carbohydrate (usually $15–30 \, gh^{-1}$ exercise) or decreasing the insulin, or both. More details about the treatment adaptation during and after exercise for the pump patient are available in Wolpert.[42]

For efforts appearing in bold in Table 2.2, insulin dosage decrease is recommended. If the activity is scheduled during the 3 h after a meal covered by a short-acting insulin analogue, it is preferable to decrease the meal bolus by 10–50 per cent. If the exercise session begins during that period but lasts for more than 3 h, it is suggested that the basal rate be decreased temporarily from 20 min prior to the effort and up to 1–3 h after the end of it. It is highly recommended to start with short exercise sessions (30 min), increase the duration progressively and check the blood glucose before, during and immediately after. Late basal rate decrease may be necessary during the night following an endurance exercise of several hours. The decrease is usually in the range of −10 to 20 per cent.

The long-acting insulin analogues

Glargine and, to a lesser extent, its cousin detemir have a duration of action that makes subtle and short duration adjustments almost impossible. It is not possible, for example, to decrease the night insulin coverage by 10 per cent without also influencing the basal insulin dose of the entire next day. If the exercise session lasts a couple of hours, it is advised to act on the meal injections before and after the effort and to snack with regular blood glucose control during the effort. An alternative solution is to split the daily long-acting analogue dose into two injections (early morning and bedtime). This allows, to a certain extent, an adjustment of the basal insulin of the day and/or the night. Smaller doses have a shorter duration of action.

Examples

Jogging for 45 min from 2.00 to 2.45 p.m.

If taking a basal/bolus regimen, the lunch (prandial) short-acting insulin (analogue or classical) would need to be reduced by 10–50 per cent. If using a twice-daily regimen of soluble and intermediate insulin, the morning dose should not be reduced because this would cause pre-lunch hyperglycaemia. In this case the only recourse would be to take extra carbohydrate.

Cycling for 45 min after dinner, from 7.00 to 7.45 p.m.

Decrease the short-acting insulin of the dinner injection (10–50 per cent) and basal night injection (10–20 per cent) for those on basal/bolus and the dinner soluble and intermediate insulins if on twice-daily injections.

Same example, pump treatment

Decrease the dinner bolus by 10–50 per cent and set the basal rate at 90 per cent from the beginning of the effort until 7:00 the next morning.

Slow swimming for 2 h from 5.00 to 7.00 pm; dinner at 7.45 p.m.

Decrease the short-acting insulin of the dinner injection (5–10 per cent × 2 = 10–20 per cent) and basal insulin of the dinner or night injection (5–10 per cent × 2 = 10–20 per cent).

Hiking or skiing from 10.00 a.m. to 01.00 p.m. and from 2.00 p.m. to 4.00 p.m. (total 5 h)

Decrease the short-acting insulins of the lunch and dinner injections (25–50 per cent) and basal insulins of the morning and evening injections (25–50 per cent).

Same example, pump treatment

Have breakfast at 6:00 a.m. Decrease the lunch and dinner bolus by 25–50 per cent each. Set the basal rate at 60 per cent during the day and 80 per cent during the night until 7:00 a.m.

In all the examples, the insulin dosage adaptations must be combined with extra carbohydrate intakes and frequent blood glucose measurements.

2.10 Conclusions

We live in a society which battles cardiovascular diseases, which are, in large part, the consequence of our lifestyles. Along with the decreased use of tobacco and healthier eating habits, regular physical exercise is of major importance for the improvement and maintenance of health.[38] In addition, exercise is a source of pleasure and social contact for many people. It is therefore only natural that strategies have been developed which permit, and even encourage, those who have type 1 diabetes to devote themselves to the physical activity of their choice.

Before undertaking any exercise programme we would advise patients to speak with their physicians and to have a general medical check-up, which should focus on the potential complications of diabetes, especially cardiovascular disease. This is even more important in those who have previously lived a sedentary lifestyle.

To be physically active, safe and confident, the diabetic person has to become familiar with certain basic rules, which we have tried to outline above. In order to learn the basic guidelines, and how to adjust one's treatment to take part in sport, contact with a team of experienced professionals is a necessity. In addition, personal experience, together with frequent blood glucose checks, permits each person to adapt the general principles to his or her own personal situation. The diabetes associations and some specific groups (see www.diabetesport.org) offer publications, workshops and classes which provide opportunities for an education in sport and diabetes and for networking with others.

References

1. American Diabetes Association. Diabetes mellitus and exercise: position statement. *Diabet Care* 1997; **20**: 1908–1912

2. Rudermann N, Devlin JT (eds), *Handbook of Exercise in Diabetes.* Alexandria, VA: American Diabetes Association, 2002.

3. Grimm JJ, Fontana E, Gremion G *et al.* Diabète de type 2: Quel exercice pour quel diabétique et comment le prescrire? In: *Journées de Diabétologie de l'Hôtel-Dieu 2004.* Paris: Flammarion Médecine-Sciences, 2004, pp. 95–104.

4. Kang J, Robertson RJ *et al.* Effect of exercise intensity on glucose and insulin metabolism in obese individuals and obese NIDDM patients. *Diabet. Care* 1996; **19**: 341–349.

5. Hagenfeldt L, Wahren J. Human forearm muscle metabolism during exercise uptake, release and oxidation of individual FFA and glycerol. *Scand. J. Clin. Lab. Invest.* 1968; **21**: 263–276.

6. Lemon PWR, Nagle FJ. Effects of exercise on protein and amino acid metabolism. *Med. Sci. Sports Exerc.* 1981; **13**: 141–149.

7. Koivisto VA. Diabetes and exercise. In: Alberti KGMM, Krall LP (eds), *The Diabetes Annual 6.* Amsterdam: Elsevier Science, 1991; pp. 169–183.

8. Moesch H, Décombaz J. In: *Nutrition et Sport* Vevey: Nestlé, 1990.

9. Wahren J, Felig P, Ahlborg G, Jorfeldt L. Glucose metabolism during leg exercise in man. *J. Clin. Invest.* 1971; **50**: 2715–2725.

10. Ahlborg G, Felig P, Hagenfeld L, Hendler R, Wahren J. Substrate turnover during prolonged exercise in man. Splanchnic and leg metabolism of glucose, FFA and amino acids. *J. Clin. Invest.* 1974; **53**: 1080–1090.

11. Stein TP, Hoyit RW, O'Toole M *et al.* Protein and energy metabolism during prolonged exercise in trained athletes. *Int. J. Sports Med.* 1989; **10**: 311–316.

12. Wasserman DH, Lacy DB, Goldstein RE, Wiliams PE, Cherrington AD. Exercise-induced fall in insulin and hepatic carbohydrate metabolism during exercise. *Am. J. Physiol.* 1989; **256**: E500–508.

13. Wasserman DH. Control of glucose fluxes during exercise in the absorptive state. *A. Rev. Physiol.* 1985; 191–218.

14. Wasserman DH, Zinnmann B. Fuel Homeostasis. In: Rudermann N, Devlin JT (eds), *The Health Professional's Guide to Diabetes and Exercise*. Alexandria: American Diabetes Association, 1995, pp. 27–47.

15. Mitchell TH, Abraham G, Schiffrin A, Leiter LA, Marliss EB. Hyperglycaemia after intense exercise in IDDM subjects during continuous subcutaneous insulin infusion. *Diabet. Care* 1988; **11**: 311–317.

16. Purdon C, Brousson M, Nyreen SL *et al*. The roles of insulin and catecholamines in the glucoregulatory response during intense exercise and early recovery in insulin-dependent diabetic and control subjects. *J. Clin. Endocinol. Metab.* 1993; **76**: 566–573.

17. Hoelzer DR, Dalsky GP, Schwartz NS *et al*. Epinephrine is not critical to prevention of hypoglycaemia during exercise in humans. *Am. J. Physiol* 1986; **251**: E104–110.

18. Wahrenberg H, Engfeldt P, Bolinder J, Arner P. Acute adaptation in adrenergic control of lipolysis during physical exercise in humans. *Am. J. Physiol.* 1987; **253**: E383–390.

19. Zinman B. Exercise in the patient with diabetes mellitus. In: Galloway JA, Potvin JH, Shuman CR (eds), *Diabetes Mellitus*. Indianapolis, IN: Lilly Research Laboratories, 1988, pp. 216–223.

20. Frid A, Linde B. Intraregional differences in the absorption of unmodified insulin from the abdominal wall. *Diabet. Med.* 1992; **9**: 236–239.

21. Vora JP. Relationship between absorption of radiolabeled soluble insulin, subcutaneous blood flow and anthropometry. *Diabet. Care* 1992; **9**: 236–239.

22. Sindelka G, Heinemann L, Berger M, Frenck W, Chantelau E. Effect of insulin concentration, subcutaneous fat thickness and skin temperature on subcutaneous insulin absorption in healthy subjects. *Diabetologia* 1994; **37**: 377–380.

23. Köhlendorf K, Bojsen J, Deckert T. Absorption and miscibility of regular porcine insulin after subcutaneous injection of insulin-treated diabetic patients. *Diabet. Care* 1983; **6**: 6–9.

24. Braak EW, Woodworth JR, Bianchi R *et al*. Injection site effects on the pharmacokinetics and glucodynamics of insulin lispro and regular insulin. *Diabet Care* 1996; **19**(12): 1437–1440.

25. Koivisto VA, Felig P. Effects of leg exercise on insulin absorption in diabetic patients. *New Engl. J. Med.* 1978; **298**: 77–83.

26. Kemmer FW, Berchtold P, Berger M *et al*. Exercise-induced fall of blood glucose in insulin-treated diabetics unrelated to alteration of insulin mobilization. *Diabetes* 1979; **28**: 1131–1137.

27. Frid A, Ostman J, Linde B. Hypoglycaemia risk during exercise after intramuscular injection of insulin in the thigh in IDDM. *Diabet. Care* 1990; **13**: 473–477.

28. Lawrence RD. The effect of exercise on insulin action in diabetes. *Br. Med. J.* 1926; **1**: 648–650.

29. McDonald MJ. Post-exercise late-onset hypoglycaemia in insulin-dependent diabetic patients. *Diabet. Care* 1987; **10**: 584–588.

30. Sonnenberg GE, Kemmer FW, Berger M. Exercise in type 1 (insulin-dependent) diabetic patients treated with continuous subcutaneous insulin infusion: prevention of exercise-induced hypoglycaemia. *Diabetologia* 1990; **33**: 696–703.

31. Amiel SA, Sherwin RS, Simonson DC, Tamborlane WV. Effect of intensive insulin therapy on glycemic thresholds for counterregulatory hormone release. *Diabetes* 1988; **37**: 901–907.

32. Berger M, Berchtold P, Cuipers HJ *et al.* Metabolic and hormonal effects of muscular exercise in juvenile type diabetes. *Diabetologia* 1977; **13**: 355–365.

33. Grimm JJ, Golay A, Habicht F, Berné C, Muchnick, S. Prevention of hypoglycaemia during exercise: more carbohydrate or less insulin? *Diabetes* 1996; **45** (suppl.): 104A (abstract).

34. Grimm JJ, Ybarra J, Berné C, Muchnick S, Golay A. A new table for prevention of hypoglycaemia during physical activity in type 1 diabetic patients. *Diabet Metab.* 2004; **30**: 465–470.

35. Tuominen JA, Karonen SL, Melamies L, Bolli G, Koivisto VA. Exercise-induced hypo-glycaemia in IDDM patients treated with a short-acting insulin analogue. *Diabetologia* 1995; **38**: 106–111.

36. Austernat E, Stahl T. *Insulinpumppentherapie.* Berlin: de Gruyter, 1989.

37. Berger W, Grimm JJ. *Insulinothérapie. Comment gérer au quotidien les variations physiologiques des besoins en insuline.* Paris: Masson, 1999.

38. Gordon NF. *Diabetes – your Complete Exercise Guide.* Champain, IL, Human Kinetics, 1993, p. 39.

39. Sane T, Helve E, Pelkonen R, Koivisto VA. The adjustment of diet and insulin dose during long-term endurance exercise in type 1 (insulin-dependent) diabetic men. *Diabetologia* 1988; **31**: 35–40.

40. Walsh J, Roberts R, Jovanovic-Peterson, L. *Stop the Rollercoaster.* San Diego, CA: Torrey Pines Press, 1996, p. 141.

41. Powell KE, Pratt M. Physical activity and health. *Br. Med. J.* 1996; **313**: 126–127.

42. Wolpert H. *Smart Pumping for People with Diabetes.* Alexandria, VA: American Diabetes Association, 2002.

43. Lepore M, Pampanelli S, Fanelli C *et al.* Pharmacokinetics and Pharmacodynamics of Subcutaneous Injection of Long-Acting Human Insulin Analog Glargine, NPH Insulin, and Ultralente Human Insulin and Continuous Subcutaneous Infusion or Insulin Lispro. *Diabetes,* **49**: 2142–2148, 2000.

3

Diet and Nutritional Strategies During Sport and Exercise in Type 1 Diabetes

Elaine Hibbert-Jones and **Gill Regan**

3.1 What is Exercise?

Exercise means different things to different people and for competitive sport involves many hours of training. For example, somebody in training for a marathon may run 30–40 miles per week; somebody participating in team sports, e.g. football, may do two 2 h sessions a week plus one competitive game a week; a recreational athlete whose main concern is their health may do 30–90 min sessions, two to four times a week.

Whatever the intensity and duration of exercise, optimum control of diabetes can only be achieved with careful planning and a good training and nutritional strategy.

3.2 The Athlete with Diabetes

Regular physical activity, diet and insulin are the cornerstones of diabetes management. The management of blood glucose levels pose a challenge for people with diabetes undertaking sport or exercise. They must have an understanding of basic food composition and know how the body regulates its fuels before, during and after exercise in order to successfully manage blood glucose levels.

Exercise and Sport in Diabetes, 2nd Edition   Edited by Dinesh Nagi
© 2005 John Wiley & Sons, Ltd.

Hypoglycaemia is a real risk to people with type 1 diabetes and especially in those taking part in hazardous sports such as water sports and rock-climbing where a 'hypo' can potentially be fatal. Hyperglycaemia can significantly affect performance, leading to fatigue. The management of blood glucose levels is therefore an important goal and having a good nutritional strategy is an essential component of exercise management.

3.3 Nutritional Principles for Optimizing Sports Performance

The International Olympic Committee (IOC) Medical Commission Working Group on Sports Nutrition has recently reviewed the key issues in sports nutrition.[1] The nutritional principles for optimizing exercise performance are very similar to the nutritional recommendations for diabetes.[2] The basic dietary requirements for energy, protein, fat, carbohydrate, vitamins and minerals are no different from a non diabetic athlete.[3] The skill is to identify when changes in insulin and/or carbohydrate are required to optimize blood glucose control for exercise, training and competition.

3.4 Putting Theory into Practice

People eat food not nutrients. The skill of a dietician is to translate the nutritional goals into an eating plan which takes into account people's food preferences and lifestyle issues. Food availability, cooking skills, financial and social considerations, timing of exercise in relation to food intake and nutritional knowledge must be considered. Athletes with type 1 diabetes need to incorporate all of these factors in combination with their current insulin regimen and predicted blood glucose response to exercise.

When planning a nutritional strategy there are two main issues to consider: first, identification of the nutritional goals and second how these goals are to be achieved in practice.

3.5 Identifying Nutritional Goals

- What are the energy requirements? Does energy intake match energy output? Are weight changes required?

- What is the macronutrient composition of the diet? Does an athlete require additional protein or need to reduce fat intake?

- Are the micronutrient needs being met, particularly iron and calcium?

- Are dietary supplements being used?

- What are the fluid requirements? Are sports drinks being used?

3.6 Energy

Energy balance is not the objective of athletic training. To maximize performance, athletes strive to achieve an optimum sports-specific body size, body composition and mix of energy stores.[4] Marathon runners require energy for endurance but do not want to carry excess body weight. Similarly, gymnasts need energy for strength but may also need to lose weight, and weight-lifters need energy to increase muscle bulk and strength.

Total energy intake must be sufficient to meet the increased energy expenditure during exercise. However, where a low body weight is advantageous or where an athlete is required to 'make weight', e.g. judo, food intake and therefore nutrient intake may be restricted. In females particularly, this can lead to problems with bone and reproductive health.

During training and competition, in sports of high intensity and long duration, the limiting factor for performance is energy intake, especially carbohydrate intake.

Key points

- The amount of energy needed depends on the intensity, duration and type of exercise undertaken.

- Total energy requirements will depend on age, sex and body weight.

- Young sports-people need additional energy for growth and development.

- Where there is a need to reduce body weight, this should be done gradually by following a sensible weight loss programme.

3.7 Carbohydrate

Carbohydrate is the most important nutrient for working muscles. It fuels the training to optimize sports performance. Carbohydrate is stored as glycogen in the liver and muscles but stores are limited. During exercise, particularly high intensity exercise such as sprint training and team sports, e.g. football, hockey, these stores are rapidly depleted. A high-carbohydrate diet, together with sufficient insulin, will ensure these stores are replenished prior to the next exercise session. If stores are not replenished, the quality of training will be sub-optimal, fatigue may occur and performance will be affected.

Carbohydrate requirements

Previous guidelines have recommended intakes of 60–70 per cent of total energy intake for athletes.[5] However, a review of dietary surveys of athletes found their intakes to be 50–55 per cent of energy.[6] It is now recommended that guidelines should be given as grams relative to body mass.[7] Carbohydrate recommendations for training are given in Table 3.1.

Table 3.1   Carbohydrate recommendations for training[8]

Level of training	Carbohydrate g/kg body weight/day
Regular (3–5 h per week)	4–5
Moderate duration/low intensity	5–7
Moderate to heavy endurance training	7–12
Extreme exercise (4–6 h per day)	10–12

Using these figures and the body weight, the total carbohydrate requirement can be calculated:

$$\text{Body weight (kg)} \quad \times \quad \frac{\text{Carbohydrate for}}{\text{level of training}} \quad = \quad \text{Total carbohydrate requirement per day}$$

$$\text{E.g. } 60 \quad \times \quad \underset{\substack{\text{(moderate duration,} \\ \text{low intensity)}}}{5\text{–}7} \quad = \quad 300\text{–}420\,\text{g day}^{-1}$$

Once the carbohydrate requirements have been estimated, suitable food choices can be made to meet these requirements. Appendix 1 gives some examples of the carbohydrate content of some foods. In addition, most food labels will have the carbohydrate content per 100 g of food (or per 100 ml if liquid) and some will give the amount per serving. However, it is important to be aware that the individual's serving size may differ from the information on the label, particularly where energy requirements are high. The total carbohydrate of the serving size will then need to be calculated.

Distribution of carbohydrate

The distribution of carbohydrate intake throughout the day will depend on the insulin regimen as well as timing of exercise, e.g.

- short-acting analogues vs human soluble insulin;

- long-acting analogues vs intermediate or long acting insulins;

- twice daily mixtures vs multiple daily injections (MDI) vs continuous sub-cutaneous insulin infusion (CSII/insulin pump therapy).

People on MDI or CSII may find it easier to control blood glucose by adjusting insulin doses to carbohydrate intake and exercise. Programmes have been developed to help to teach people the skills they need to do this.[9,10]

Low or high glycaemic index?

The glycaemic index (GI) is used as a measure of how quickly foods that contain carbohydrate raise blood glucose levels. The greater the rise in blood glucose, the higher the GI value. Generally foods are grouped under three categories: low, moderate and high. Foods with a high GI tend to cause a sharp rise in blood glucose levels. Low GI foods produce a more gentle rise in blood glucose levels.

Although a variety of tables of GI values for food have been published, they can only be used as a guide. This is because the GI can be affected by a number of factors, e.g. variety, brand, country of origin, method of cooking, degree of processing and the content of the previous meal. A food could have a high rating in one table and a moderate rating in another.

Studies in non-diabetic athletes found greater glycogen storage during 24 h post-recovery when high GI foods were consumed.[11] In people with diabetes, the total amount of carbohydrate has a much greater influence on glycaemia than the source or type of carbohydrate.[2] More research is required before recommendations can be made on the use of GI, particularly as the majority of current evidence is based on studies with non-diabetic, non-exercising individuals.

3.8   Guidelines for Carbohydrate Intake Before, During and After Exercise

Before exercise

The blood glucose level should be monitored. What should the target level of blood glucose be before exercise?

- Avoid exercise if blood glucose level is $>14\,\mathrm{mmol\,l^{-1}}$ $(250\,\mathrm{mg\,dl^{-1}})$ and ketones are present.

- Exercise with caution if blood glucose level is $>17\,\mathrm{mmol\,l^{-1}}$ $(>300\,\mathrm{mg\,dl^{-1}})$ without ketones.

- Take extra carbohydrate if blood glucose level is $<5.5\,\mathrm{mmol\,l^{-1}}$ $(100\,\mathrm{mg\,dl^{-1}})$.[12]

Additional carbohydrate for exercise

The rigid recommendation to use carbohydrate supplementation, calculated from the planned intensity and duration of physical activity, without regard to the glycaemic level at the start of the activity, the previous metabolic response and the patient's insulin therapy, is no longer appropriate. The dietitian's advice therefore needs to be tailored to the needs of the individual, taking into consideration the above recommendations.

Role of insulin

The amount of insulin circulating before, during and after exercise and the blood glucose level is critical to exercise performance and prevention of fatigue (Table 3.2).

Table 3.2 Blood glucose response and circulating insulin levels

Status of plasma insulin	Hepatic glucose production	Muscle glucose utilisation	Blood glucose
Normal or slightly diminished	↑	↑	→
Markedly diminished	↑	↗	↗
Increased	↗	↑	↓

Reproduced courtesy of the Sugar Bureau in association with the British Olympic Association.

- Too much insulin circulating during exercise will inhibit hepatic glucose production and increase blood glucose uptake by the muscles, leading to hypoglycaemia.

- Too little insulin circulating during exercise may cause blood glucose levels to increase due to hepatic glucose production and a reduction in blood glucose uptake by the muscles.

- If ketones are present, exercise may contribute to diabetic ketoacidosis.

Role of carbohydrate

- A high carbohydrate meal should be eaten 2–3 h before exercise.

- Additional carbohydrate *may* be needed 20–30 min before exercise depending on the pre-exercise blood glucose level, the type and duration of exercises and the normal response to the exercise. This may be provided by fluid or food containing rapidly absorbed carbohydrate, e.g. isotonic sports drink, fruit juice, glucose tablets, confectionery, cereal bar, fruit.

- It is not possible to make specific recommendations for the quantity of additional carbohydrate needed because of the many factors that can affect the athlete's glucose response to exercise. Recently, Grimm *et al.* have proposed a table of carbohydrate supplementation, to prevent hypoglycaemia, for physical activity of different intensity and duration. However, it is designed for patients who have good metabolic control during the hours before exercise[12]. More research is needed in this area.

During exercise

The blood glucose level should be monitored when practical.

- Hypoglycaemia may develop during exercise because of the increased glucose uptake by the working muscles or because there is too much insulin circulating.

- For exercise lasting more than 30 min, extra carbohydrate may be needed and/or insulin reduced.

- Pre-exercise sources of carbohydrate may also be useful during exercise, but practical considerations such as availability, abdominal discomfort and rules ofthe sport will influence both choice of carbohydrate and timing of intake.

- A hypo remedy must be available and accessible at all times.

After exercise – refuelling

The blood glucose level should be monitored.

- The highest rates of muscle glycogen repletion occur in the first hour after exercise.

- Immediately after exercise (0–4 h) consume 1.0–1.2 g carbohydrate at frequent intervals.[7]

- Failure to consume carbohydrate in this time leads to low rates of glycogen refuelling.

- This is particularly important when there are only 4–6 h between training sessions. Snacks containing carbohydrate with a high GI may be better tolerated during this time because of reduced appetite post exercise.

- Snacks containing carbohydrate with a high GI are best consumed during this time.

- When longer recovery periods are available, athletes can choose when to eat. The total carbohydrate consumed appears to be more important than the pattern of intake.[7]

- Muscle damage interferes with glycogen storage – this may be partially offset by an increased carbohydrate intake in the first 24 h of recovery.

- Insulin is required for the refuelling process for athletes with type 1 diabetes. If there is insufficient circulating insulin, less glycogen can be stored and this may affect future training and exercise sessions.

- Muscle glycogen stores can be enhanced by the addition of protein provided that the supplementation is within 1 h.[13] When the athlete's energy intake or food availability does not allow them to consume sufficient carbohydrate, the presence of protein in the post-exercise meals and snacks may enhance overall glycogen recovery.[7]

- Post exercise-induced hypoglycaemia can develop some hours after the end of the exercise session as glycogen is resynthesized from circulating blood glucose. A combination of adjustment of carbohydrate intake and insulin, in response to blood glucose levels, will help to reduce the risk of hypoglycaemia.

- Low GI foods can be consumed in the recovery period. Table 3.3 lists some useful ideas for snacks for the kitbag.

Table 3.3   Kitbag snacks

- Dried fruit, e.g. raisins, apricots, fruit and nut mix.
- Scones, muffins, teacakes, fruit bread.
- Fruit cake, scotch pancakes, Jaffa Cakes.
- Cereal bars, rice cakes, popcorn.
- Biscuits, confectionery, e.g. jelly beans, fruit pastilles.
- Sandwiches, rolls, pitta bread (with low-fat fillings).
- Fresh fruit, individual tins of fruit.
- Milk, low-fat yoghurt, fromage frais.
- Low-fat crisps and snacks.

Key points

- Aim to achieve carbohydrate intakes to meet energy requirements for training and refuelling glycogen stores between exercise sessions.

- The highest rates of muscle glycogen repletion occur in the first hour after exercise.

- Consume some protein with carbohydrate-rich snacks post-exercise.

- Carbohydrate can be taken as food or fluid.

- Ensure an adequate energy intake and sufficient insulin to optimize blood glucose levels and glycogen resynthesis.

- Avoid excessive consumption of alcohol after exercise. It can interfere with the athlete's ability to eat sensibly after exercise and increases the risk of hypoglycaemia.

3.9 Protein

Most athletes have enough protein in their normal diet to meet the needs of training, providing that the energy intake is adequate (Table 3.4).[14] Individuals with diabetes have been found to consume around 1.5 g protein kg^{-1} body weight per day or 10–20 per cent of energy.[15] The American Diabetes Association recommends that people with diabetes avoid intakes greater than 20 per cent of energy because the long-term effects of consuming this amount on the development of nephropathy have not been determined.[16] Diabetes UK have recommended no more than 1 g kg^{-1} body weight per day.[2]

Table 3.4 Sources of protein in the diet

Animal (tend to be higher in saturated fat)	Vegetable (tend to be higher in carbohydrate/fibre)
Meat, poultry, offal	Pulses (peas, beans, lentils)
Fish, shellfish	TVP (textured vegetable protein)
Cheese	Tofu, Quorn
Eggs	Nuts, seeds
Milk	Soya products
Yoghurt	

Protein requirements for athletes

Endurance athletes need sufficient protein to maintain lean body mass and not impair performance. In strength and team sports protein is required to increase muscle mass for strength and power. It is the exercise training which brings about the adaptations in the muscle, not the amount of protein consumed.

Previously, recommendations have been made for protein intakes for athletes:

- Strength or speed athletes, 1.2–1.7 g protein kg^{-1} body weight per day;

- Endurance athletes, 1.2–1.4 g protein kg^{-1} body weight per day.[17]

However, most athletes are already eating 1.2–1.7 g protein kg^{-1} body weight per day and so 'additional' protein is not required.[18] For a 70 kg person this would equate to 84–120 g protein per day. Tables A2 and A3 in the Appendix show the amount of protein in food portions.

Other factors can also affect the usage of ingested protein and amino acids:

- Type of protein – essential amino acids stimulate muscle protein synthesis. Only animal protein contains all the essential amino acids. A good mixture of the vegetable proteins must be eaten to ensure a sufficient intake of essential amino acids.

- Adding carbohydrate to a source of amino acids can improve the response of muscle protein balance following exercise.

- Timing of protein intake and ingestion with carbohydrate can also have an effect. This is discussed more fully by Tipton and Wolfe.[14]

Key points

- Most athletes consume enough protein in their normal diet to meet the additional needs of training.

- Many protein foods are also high in fat, so wise choices need to be made (Table 3.4).

- People with additional dietary restrictions, e.g. vegetarians, may still meet their protein needs providing suitable food choices are made.

- Protein and amino acid supplements are not normally necessary.

3.10   Fat

Fat is an essential nutrient in the diet. The recommendations for people with diabetes are:

- limit total fat to <35 per cent energy intake;

- limit saturated fat to <10 per cent energy;

- use monounsaturated fats as the main fat source, together with ω-3 polyun-saturated fat.[2]

Unlike glycogen, there is always sufficient fat available as fuel for exercise, even in the leanest of competitors. It was therefore assumed that fat played no part in enhancing performance. However, there has been interest in intramuscular tri-acylglycerol (IMTG), which provides a potentially important energy source for the contracting muscle[19] and its repletion following exercise. This is discussed by Spriet and Gibala,[20] but currently there is insufficient evidence to identify strategies which enhance adaptations to training.

For most athletes with diabetes, reducing total fat to ensure sufficient carbohy-drate is the main goal. This can be achieved by making suitable food choices and using low fat cooking methods.

3.11 Vitamin and Minerals

For athletes consuming a varied, balanced diet which meets their energy needs, there is no evidence that vitamin and mineral supplementation is necessary to enhance health or performance. Excessive intakes may be harmful. There are, however, some situations in which qualified medical practitioners, accredited sports dietitians and registered nutritionists may recommend specific vitamins or minerals for certain individuals, e.g. if iron stores are low. These should only be taken as directed or prescribed. Caution is needed because there is no guarantee that vitamin and mineral supplements are free from prohibited substances.[21] This could be important for top-level athletes.

Supplements

The use of dietary supplements in sport is widespread. A well-balanced diet that meets the energy demands of training should provide the athlete with all the essential nutrients.

Informed dietary choices can ensure full needs are met to promote:

- adaptation to training;

- recovery from training;

- improvements in health, reducing illness and injury.

Special sports foods, such as energy bars, sports drinks and carbohydrate gels may have a role to play, especially in maintaining blood glucose levels within the target range during exercise. Protein supplements and meal replacements may be useful in some situations. Where there is a demonstrated deficiency of an essential nutrient, an increase from food or supplementation may be necessary. However many athletes take supplements in doses that are not necessary or may even be harmful.[22]

Some supplements do offer the possibility of increasing performance; these include creatine, caffeine, bicarbonate and possibly a few others, but as a result of poor manufacturing some supplements have been shown to contain impurities, including anabolic androgenic steroids.

Nutritional supplements are not generally subject to regulation by the Food and Drug Administration (FDA). Athletes are therefore unable to accurately determine what ingredients supplements contain or how pure the product is.

Athletes who are liable for dope testing under national or international programmes should be extra cautious about supplement usage. In addition the principle of strict liability applies, which means the athlete is responsible for all food and drink consumed.

Key point

It is recommended that strategies for the inclusion of dietary supplements should be discussed in consultation with the diabetes team. This is due to the range of supplements available, possible side effects, the effect on diabetes control and issues relating to contamination.

3.12   Fluid and Hydration

Most exercise sessions result in some degree of sweating leading to a loss of water and salts. Fluid replacement is required to maintain hydration and allow the athlete to perform and limit fatigue. Inadequate fluid intake will adversely affect temperature regulation, cardiovascular function and muscle metabolism.

Fluid requirements

In general sedentary people need about 2–3 l of fluid per day to remain fully hydrated. Sweat rates during exercise are typically $0.5–1.5 \, l \, h^{-1}$,[23] but can increase in trained individuals up to $3 \, l \, h^{-1}$ in hot and humid conditions. During exercise it is important to limit dehydration by drinking fluids at a rate that most closely matches sweating rate. However, because sweat rates vary greatly between individuals and the fluid requirements will also be influenced by fitness levels and duration of exercise, the best advice is to measure body weight loss by weighing the athlete before and after exercise.

- 1 kg weight loss represents approximately 1 l of sweat loss;

- a weight loss of greater than 2 per cent, especially when exercising in a hot and humid environment (>30 °C), is likely to impair exercise performance;

- 2 per cent weight loss equates to 1 kg for a 50 kg person, 1.5 kg for a 75 kg person and 2 kg for a 100 kg person.

Fluid intake should be sufficient to replace total sweat losses. Avoid excess fluid intake during exercise to prevent an increase in body weight. Fluid lost is estimated at 1.2–1.5 times the actual fluid lost during exercise to allow for obligatory losses e.g. continued sweating and urine production.

When it is not possible to weigh before and after exercise, another good indicator of fluid loss is to determine the volume and colour of urine produced. Pale and plentiful urine generally indicates the athlete is hydrated; dark and sparse urine is an indication that more fluid is required.

Key point

Dehydration can lead to a rise in body temperature, light-headedness, nausea, fatigue or heatstroke and must not be confused with symptoms of hypoglycaemia.

Fluid intake and exercise

Drinking plenty of fluids to avoid compromising health as well as to improve exercise performance is essential. To succeed, it is important to plan drinking strategies for the athlete and to recommend they practise drinking during exercise so that the body can adapt to the necessary fluid intake required for the planned level of exercise.

Guidelines for fluid replacement before, during and after exercise

Before exercise

Blood glucose should be monitored before exercise.

- Always start an exercise session fully hydrated. Thirst is a poor indicator of hydration status.

- Drinking 400–600 ml water in the 2 h before exercise will help hydrate the body.[24] Sports drinks containing carbohydrate need to be used with caution because of the effect they may have on the pre-exercise blood glucose level. However, they may be useful to maintain blood glucose levels within the target range during exercise. This range needs to be agreed with the diabetes team.

- Water, no-added-sugar squash, regular squash and isotonic sports drinks can all be useful, depending upon the intensity and duration of the exercise, the blood glucose level and the environmental conditions in which it takes place.

- Sports drinks containing carbohydrate may also be useful for the correction of hypoglycaemia.

During exercise

Blood glucose levels should be monitored during exercise where possible.

- Aim to drink enough fluid to limit losses as sweat. Drinking small volumes frequently will minimize gastric discomfort.

- During exercise lasting more than 1 h athletes are advised to drink 150–200 ml fluid every 15–20 mins (30–60 g carbohydrate/h) to offset fluid losses. The choice of fluid will depend on the athlete's strategy for maintaining blood glucose levels within the target range during exercise.

- Sports drinks containing 6–8 g carbohydrate 100 ml^{-1} may be useful in providing both carbohydrate and fluid to maintain both blood glucose levels and hydration during the exercise period.

- Sodium should be included in fluids consumed during exercise for more than 2 h. Isotonic sports drinks generally contain added electrolytes.

- Drinking excessively during exercise resulting in weight gain is not recommended.

- Caffeine taken during the later stages of exercise when taken in quantities of 1.5 mg kg^{-1} has been found to be ergogenic.

- No benefit is gained from the ingestion of glycerol and amino acid supplements during exercise.

After exercise

Blood glucose levels should be monitored after exercise.

- Complete restoration of fluid balance after exercise is an important part of the recovery process.

- Fluid replacement will be dependent on how much fluid has been lost during exercise.

- The volume of fluid taken should be greater than the volume of fluid lost to allow for the ongoing obligatory losses, e.g. sweat and urine.

- Research shows that athletes drink larger volumes when the drink is flavoured.

- Isotonic sports drinks containing 4–8 per cent (4–8 g 100 ml^{-1}) carbohydrate may be useful for maintaining post-exercise blood glucose levels and refuelling glycogen stores after exercise. Sufficient insulin must be available for the refuelling process.

- Rehydration after exercise requires not only the replacement of volume losses but also the replacement of electrolytes, primarily sodium lost in sweat. This can be achieved by adding salt to food or eating salty snacks. Salt supplements are not normally necessary.

Sports drinks

The composition of sports drinks is a key factor for consideration in terms of beverage choice when used for fluid replacement before, during and after exercise. Most sports drinks aim to influence performance by providing the athlete with both a fluid and energy source from carbohydrate. The carbohydrate is generally derived from sugars (glucose, sucrose and fructose), maltodextrins or other rapidly absorbed carbohydrates.

The formulation of sports drinks is generally classified as hypotonic, isotonic or hypertonic (Table 3.5). The rate of fluid delivery to the body depends on the composition of the drink, which influences, how much is drunk, how quickly it is emptied from the stomach and how quickly it is absorbed from the intestine. Studies have shown that sports drinks are an efficient way to supply both fluid and fuel. The choice of sports drink used will depend on the athlete's priority for fluid or fuel and the maintenance of blood glucose levels within the target range before, during and after exercise.

Table 3.5   Composition of different types of sports drinks

Type of drink	Carbohydrate concentration, g $100\,ml^{-1}$	Dissolved substances, e.g. glucose/electrolytes	Fluid or fuel replacement	Effect on blood glucose level
Hypotonic	<4 g	Low	Fluid	↑ or →
Isotonic	4–8 g	Same as body fluids	Fluid and fuel	↑↑
Hypertonic	>8 g	High	Fuel	↑↑↑

Water vs sports drinks

The choice between water and sports drinks, as fluid replacement, will be dependent on the following factors:

- pre- and post-exercise blood glucose levels;

- timing and availability of circulating insulin;

- duration and intensity of exercise;

- environmental conditions, e.g. heat, humidity and cold;

- training status, i.e. fitness;

- strategies for fluid replacement before, during and after exercise need to be made with the athlete in consultation with their diabetes team, taking into account the type and duration of exercise that is to be undertaken.

Key points

- Fluid intake is essential during exercise.

- Start exercise fully hydrated.

- Athletes tend to drink too little rather than too much.

- Thirst is a poor indicator of hydration status. Athletes should drink before they are thirsty to ensure adequate fluid intake.

- Flavoured drinks may encourage greater fluid intake than plain water. Ensure availability of palatable drinks.

- Avoid carbonated drinks which may cause gastric disturbances.

- Start rehydration immediately after exercise.

- Ensure a high-carbohydrate drink is always available for treatment and correction of hypoglycaemia.

3.13   Pulling It All Together

A number of factors need to be considered when developing a nutritional strategy for sport and exercise:

- Is the exercise planned or unplanned? Unplanned exercise usually requires additional carbohydrate. Adjustments can be made to insulin prior to planned exercise which may reduce the amount of additional carbohydrate which needs to be consumed.

- Type of exercise – different types of exercise will have different nutritional requirements and different effects on the blood glucose level, e.g. resistance training such as weight-lifting, endurance exercise such as running, high-intensity exercise such as sprinting, intermittent, high intensity exercise such as ball games.

- Pre-exercise blood glucose level and the athlete's usual response to different types of exercise.

- Timing of exercise in relation to timing of both insulin and carbohydrate intake.

- Duration and intensity of exercise.

- Training status, e.g. fitness level.

- Frequency and length of time between exercise sessions.

- Environmental factors, e.g. humidity, temperature (hot and cold).

- Hydration status – the perceived effort will be greater in an athlete who is poorly hydrated.

- Clothing – additional clothing worn for exercise may cause an increase in sweating rates.

- Team sports – position played, strength of opposition.

- Competitive athletes will need a different nutritional strategy prior to competition. This needs to be tried and tested in low-key events.

Key points

- Monitor blood glucose levels before, during and after exercise.

- Avoid exercise if blood glucose levels before exercise are >14 mmol with ketones and use caution if levels are >17 mmol without ketones. Take extra carbohydrate if blood glucose level is <5.5 mmol.

- Encourage people with diabetes to learn their own blood glucose response to different types of exercise.

- Identify when changes in insulin and/or carbohydrate intake are necessary.

- People with diabetes who regularly participate in sport may find it useful to keep a record of carbohydrate intake, details of exercise sessions, insulin doses and blood glucose levels.

- Ensure an adequate fluid intake.

- Keep a hypo remedy *readily* available at all times.

- It is essential that people with diabetes are encouraged to discuss their individual insulin regimens and dietary requirements with their diabetes team.

Additional Information

The rigid recommendation to use carbohydrate supplementation, calculated from the planned intensity and duration of physical activity, without regard to the glycaemic level at the start of the activity, the previous metabolic response and the patient's insulin therapy, is no longer appropriate.

Recently Grimm *et al.* have proposed a table of carbohydrate supplementation, to prevent hypoglycaemia, for physical activity of different intensity and duration. However, it is designed for patients who have good metabolic control during the hours before exercise (13). More research is needed in this area.

References

1. International Olympic Committee. Sports nutrition. *J Sports Sci* 2004; **22**(1): 1–146.
2. Diabetes UK. The implementation of nutritional advice for people with diabetes. *Diab Med* 2003; **20**: 786–807.
3. Colberg S. *The Diabetic Athlete*. Leeds: Human Kinetics, 2001.
4. Loucks AB. Energy balance and body composition in sports and exercise. *J Sports Sci* 2004; **22**: 1–14.
5. Devlin JT, Williams C (eds). Final consensus statement: foods, nutrition and sports performance. *J Sports Sci* 1991; **9** (suppl.): iii.
6. Burke LM, Cox GR, Cummings NK, Desbrow B. Guidelines for daily carbohydrate intake: do athletes achieve them? *Sports Med* 2001; **31**: 267–299.
7. Burke LM, Kiens B, Ivy JL. Carbohydrates and fat for training and recovery. *J Sports Sci* 2004; **22**: 15–30.
8. Stear S. Fuelling training and recovery. In *Fuelling Fitness for Sports Performance*. The Sugar Bureau, 2004; 33–51.
9. DAFNE Study Group. Training in flexible intensive insulin management to enable dietary freedom in people with type 1 diabetes: Dose Adjustment for Normal Eating (DAFNE) randomised controlled trial. *Br Med J* 2002; **325**: 746–749.
10. Everett J, Jenkins E, Kerr D, Cavan DA. Implementation of an effective outpatient intensive education programme for patients with type 1 diabetes. *Pract Diabet Int* 2003; **20**(2): 51–55.
11. Burke LM, Collier GR, Hargreaves M. Muscle glycogen storage after prolonged exercise: the effect of glycaemic index of carbohydrate feedings. *J Appl Physiol* 1993; **75**: 1019–1023.
12. Grimm JJ, Ybarra J, Berné C, Muchnick S, Golay A. A new table for prevention of hypoglycaemia during physical activity in type 1 diabetic patients. *Diabetes Metab* 2004; **30**: 465–470.
13. Ivy JL, Gosforth HW, Damon BD, McCauley TR, Parsons EC, Price TB. Early post-exercise muscle glycogen recovery is enhanced with a carbohydrate-protein supplement. *J Appl Physiol* 2002; **93**: 1337–1344.
14. Tipton KD, Wolfe RR. Protein and amino acids for athletes. *J Sports Sci* 2003; **22**(1): 65–79.
15. Ha TKK, Lean MEJ. Technical review. Recommendations for the nutritional management of patients with diabetes mellitus. *Eur J Clin Nutr* 1998; **52**: 467–481.
16. American Diabetes Association. Evidence-based nutritional principles and recommendations for the treatment and prevention of diabetes and related complications. *Diabetes Care* 2003; **26**: S51–S61.
17. Lemon PW. Effect of exercise on protein requirements. *J Sports Sci* 1991; **9**: S3–S70.
18. Stear S. The protein question. In *Fuelling Fitness for Sports Performance*. The Sugar Bureau, 2004; 53–65.
19. Watt MJ, Heigenhauser GJF, Spriet LL. IMTG utilisation in human skeletal muscle during exercise: is there a controversy? *J Appl Physiol* 2002; **93**: 1185–1195.
20. Spriet LL, Gibala MJ. Nutritional strategies to influence adaptations to training. *J Sports Sci* 2004; **22**: 127–141.
21. UK Sport, British Olympic Association (BOA), British Paralympic Association (BPA), National Sports Medicine Institute (NSMI) and Home Country Sports Councils (HCSC). Position statement. Advice to UK athletes on the use of supplements, 2003; www.mpagb. org.uk/notices/supplements.pdf (accessed September 2004).
22. Maughan RJ, King DS, Lea T. Dietary supplements. *J Sports Sci* 2004; **22**: 95–113.
23. Maughan R. Eating for exercise. *Nutr Pract* 2004; **5**(2): 1–3.
24. Shirreffs SM, Armstrong LE, Cheuuvront SN. Fluid and electrolyte needs for preparation and recovery from training and competition. *J Sports Sci* 2004; **22**: 57–63.
25. Coyle EF. Fluid and fuel intake during exercise. *J Sports Sci* 2004; **22**: 39–55.

Appendices

Table A1   Carbohydrate content of common food items

Description of food	Approximate weight of portion (g)	Typical portion size	Carbohydrate per portion (g)	Carbohydrate per 100 g
Bakery products				
Croissant	60 g	1	23	38
Crumpet	40 g	1 round	15	39
Currant bun	60 g	1	30	53
French bread baguette	120 g	15 cm slice	65	55
Fruit scone	50 g	1	25	53
Malted grain roll	58 g	1	27	46
Malt loaf	35 g	1 slice	20	57
Naan bread	75 g	Small	55	50
	160 g	Large	80	50
Pitta bread	75 g	Small	45	58
Tortilla (wheat)	63 g	1 wrap	30	48
White bread (large loaf)	30 g	1 medium slice	15	50
	40 g	1 thick slice	20	50
White soft roll	45 g	1	25	52
Wholemeal bread (large loaf)	35 g	1 medium slice	15	42
	45 g	1 thick slice	20	42
Biscuits				
Cream crackers	15 g	2	10	70
Fig roll	20 g	1	10	50
Jaffa cake	13 g	1	9	68
Oatcake	15 g	1	10	63
Plain digestive	15 g	1	10	70
Rice cakes	15 g	1	12	75
Rye crispbread	20 g	2	15	70
Breakfast cereals				
Bran flakes	30 g	Small bowl	20	69
Cornflakes	30 g	Small bowl	25	86
Muesli (including no-added-sugar varieties)	50 g	5 tablespoons	33	66
Porridge with milk	150 g	Small bowl	20	14
Shredded wheat	22.5 g	1	15	68
Shreddies	45 g	Small bowl	30	74
Special K	30 g	Small bowl	25	81
Weetabix	20 g	1	15	76
Cereal bar	33 g	1 bar	20	65
Pasta and rice				
Couscous		$\frac{1}{2} \times 100$ g sachet, made up	38	29

(continued)

Table A.1 Continued

Description of food	Approximate weight of portion (g)	Typical portion size	Carbohydrate per portion (g)	Carbohydrate per 100 g
Pasta (cooked)				
average adult portion	220 g	5 tablespoons	50	22
Pasta (uncooked)	75 g		55	74
Quick noodles (uncooked)	90 g	1 packet	60	67
Rice				
Average adult portion	180 g	5 tablespoons	55	30
Express rice	250 g	1 packet	75	30
Tinned ravioli	220 g	$\frac{1}{2}$ large can	22	10
Tinned spaghetti	220 g	$\frac{1}{2}$ large can	30	14
Potatoes				
Boiled	60 g	1 average	10	17
Crisps	30 g	1 packet	15	53
Jacket	180 g	1 medium	60	32
Mashed	60 g	1 scoop	10	16
New boiled in skin	40 g	1 average	6	15
Oven chips	50 g	6–8 chips	15	30
Roast	50 g	1 small	15	26
Waffle (large)	45 g	1	15	30
Pulses				
Baked beans	135 g	$\frac{1}{3}$ large can	20 g	15
Chick peas (canned)	60 g	2 tablespoons	10	16
Red kidney beans (canned)	60 g	2 tablespoons	10	18
Sweetcorn kernels	50 g	2 tablespoons	10	20
Fruit				
Apple	100 g	1 small	12	12
Banana (with skin)	135 g	1 medium	20	15
Dried apricots	25 g	3	10	43
Grapes	60 g	12 grapes	10	15
Raisins	30 g	1 heaped tablespoon	20	70
Drinks				
Fruit juice	100 ml	1 small glass	10	9–10
Isotonic drink	330 ml	1 can	20	6
Lucozade Energy	50 ml		10	17

Table A2   Food portions providing 20 g of animal protein

Food item	Approximate weight (g)	Handy measure
Meat	75	2 medium slices
Poultry	75	1 small chicken breast
Fish	100	1 small fillet/1 small can
Fish fingers	100	6 fingers
Eggs	180	3 medium
Cheese	75 g	2 matchbox size pieces
Milk	600 ml	1 pint
Yoghurt	400	3 pots

Table A3   Food portions providing 10 g of vegetable protein

Food item	Approximate weight (g)	Handy measure
Nuts	50	1 medium packet
Seeds, e.g. sunflower, sesame	50	4 tablespoons
Baked beans	200	4 tablespoons
Lentils	150	5 tablespoons
Hummus	125	3 tablespoons
Tofu	125	$\frac{1}{2}$ packet
Quorn	100	
Soya milk	350 ml	Approx $\frac{2}{3}$ pint

4

The Role of Physical Activity in the Prevention of Type 2 Diabetes

Dinesh Nagi

4.1 Exercise and Prevention of Type 2 Diabetes

The prevalence of diabetes is rising rapidly worldwide, and certain developing nations are currently going through an upsurge of type 2 diabetes of epidemic proportions.[1] This is likely to have huge socio-economic consequences for healthcare resources in these countries due to considerable expense associated with complications of type 2 diabetes.[2] Primary prevention of type 2 diabetes is, therefore, of particular interest to health economists as it has in-built secondary and tertiary prevention of complications related to diabetes. This chapter is not meant to be a comprehensive review of prevention of diabetes, but will deal mostly with the results of recently published randomized trials, which have used lifestyle intervention, including physical activity, to reduce or prevent type 2 diabetes.

However, we must remember that these studies were performed in subjects at high risk of future diabetes and not in those with normal glucose tolerance. Therefore findings of these trials may not be applicable to the population at large. Therefore, in any community-based or public health approach to prevent diabetes and related diseases such as coronary heart disease, this is important for effective utilization of resources.

Type 2 diabetes has a number of disease characteristics which make it potentially a preventable disease.[3,4] Considerable knowledge exists about risk factors for diabetes which are potentially modifiable.[5] Although there is a strong genetic predisposition to this disease, environmental factors play an important role in the development of clinical diabetes. It is also clear that both insulin resistance and defective insulin secretion contribute to the development of diabetes, although

Exercise and Sport in Diabetes, 2nd Edition   Edited by Dinesh Nagi
© 2005 John Wiley & Sons, Ltd.

the relative contribution of each of these two components varies in different populations and individuals within a population.[6–8]

In most subjects predisposed to develop type 2 diabetes, there is generally a long but variable period during which minor degree of glucose intolerance exists.[9–12] This stage of pre-diabetes can be recognized by performing an oral glucose tolerance test and is known as impaired glucose tolerance (IGT). It can also be diagnosed by measuring fasting plasma glucose, known as impaired fasting glucose (IFG).[13,1] Subjects thus identified are at a higher risk of future diabetes compared with those whose glucose tolerance is normal.[9–12] Identification of subjects at high risk of diabetes provides us with an opportunity to modify the disease process, either to delay or prevent it from becoming clinically manifest.

As in type 2 diabetes, insulin resistance and defective insulin secretion contribute to the development of IGT and IFG. Both of these defects can be modified through lifestyle interventions and/or pharmacological therapies.[3] In spite of this, it has only recently been shown that type 2 diabetes can be prevented.[15] Behaviour modification through diet and exercise are attractive and have the added advantage of modifying other associated conditions such as coronary artery disease, hypertension and obesity.[16] However, lifestyle modifications are extremely difficult to sustain over the lifetime of a given individual. In addition, it is likely that different strategies may need to be adopted in different ethnic groups to improve adherence to measures which will promote healthy lifestyles.[17]

It has been known for some time that physical inactivity is associated with increased risk of type 2 diabetes. The results of various epidemiological and observational studies are summarized in Table 4.1 and showed that regular physical activity had a protective effect on the development of type 2 diabetes. These studies were remarkable for their consistent findings in the protective effects of physical activity on the occurrence of type 2 diabetes. In addition, some of the studies also showed a dose–response relationship between the frequency of physical activity and the degree of protective effect.[18–22] These studies suggested a causative role for physical inactivity in type 2 diabetes.

Table 4.1 Prospective studies of physical activity and risk of type 2 diabetes

Study population	Reference	Follow-up	Sex	Protective effect of exercise
Physician Health Study	18	5 years	Men	Yes
US College Alumni	19	Variable	Women	Yes
Pennsylvania Alumni	24	14 years	Men	Yes
Nurses' Health Study	20	8 years	Women	Yes
Malmo Study	23	6 years	Men	Yes

In the Physician Health Study published by Manson et al.,[18] 21 271 males were followed over a 5 year period. In this study, the incidence of diabetes was negatively related to the frequency of exercise (369 cases per 100 000 person-years in those who exercised less than once a week and 214 in those who exercised more than five times a week). The age-adjusted risk of diabetes in men who exercised at least once a week was 0.64 compared to those who exercised less frequently. The protective effect of exercise was unrelated to baseline body mass index (BMI) and was more marked in obese subjects.

In the study by Helmrich et al.,[19] type 2 diabetes was observed in 202 subjects out of 5990 male subjects. In this study, leisure time physical activity, expressed as number of calories expended was found to be inversely related to development of diabetes. The age-adjusted risk of diabetes was 6 per cent lower for each 500 kcal expended. These beneficial effects of exercise remained significant when adjusted for the confounding effects of obesity, blood pressure and parental history of diabetes.

In the Nurses Health Study, women who participated in vigorous physical activity at least once a week had a 33 per cent lower risk of diabetes compared with those who did not take part in such activities.[20] No dose–response relationship between frequency of exercise and risk of diabetes was seen in this study.

In the Honolulu Heart Study, subjects were followed for a period of 6 years and the cumulative incidence of diabetes was lower with increasing levels of physical activity in both men and women.[21] The age-adjusted odds ratio for diabetes comparing subjects who were in the upper quintile with those in the lower four quintile was 0.55 for men and 0.50 in women, i.e. in both men and women in the highest quintile of physical activity the risk of diabetes was approximately half compared with the rest.

A study recently published by Lynch et al.,[22] in 897 middle-aged Finnish men, showed that, self reported moderate intensity exercise undertaken for 40 min per week was associated with 56 per cent lower risk of type 2 diabetes. They also found that high levels of cardiorespiratory physical fitness (O_2 consumption in a respiratory chamber) also had a protective effect on the development of diabetes. In subjects who were at high risk of diabetes, with even a moderate degree of physical activity taken once a week for more than 40 min, the risk of diabetes was 64 per cent lower than those who did not take part in physical activity.

These studies were observational and formed the basis for conducting well-designed, randomized clinical trials to assess the effects of interventions incorporating physical activity on future development of type 2 diabetes. The major concern in the use of lifestyle intervention to prevent diabetes has been around the issue of long-term sustainability of this intervention. The study by Eriksson et al.,[23] which is discussed in Chapter 5, showed that it was possible for subjects to comply with a behaviour modification for up to 6 years, with good outcomes even after a 12 year follow-up.

These major intervention trails published over the last few years are summarized in Table 4.2. The Da-Qing study from China was the first population-based

Table 4.2 Intervention studies to reduce incidence of type 2 diabetes

Name	Number of subjects	Characteristics of subjects	Mean duration (years)	Intervention	Incidence of diabetes (% per annum)
Diabetes Prevention Programme (USA)	3234	IGT	2.8	Control	11.0
				lifestyle[a]	4.8
				Metformin	7.8
Diabetes Prevention Study (Finland)	522	IGT	3.2	Control	7.8
				lifestyle[b]	3.2
Da-Qing IGT and Diabetes Study (China)	577	IGT	6	Control	13.3
				diet[c]	8.3
				Exercise[d]	5.1
				Diet and exercise	6.8
STOP-NIDDM Acarbose Study (multinational)	1429	IGT	3.3	Placebo	12.1
				Acarbose	9.7
TRIPOD (USA)	236	Previous GDM	2.5	Placebo	12.1
				Troglitazone	5.4

[a]At least 7 per cent weight loss and 150 min physical exercise activity per week.
[b]At least 5 per cent weight loss and 210 min physical exercise activity per week.
[c]Target BMI of 23.
[d]Increase exercise by at least 1 unit per day (e.g. extra 30 min of slow walking or 5 min of swimming).

randomized study. In this study 576 subjects with IGT were randomized as to diet alone, exercise alone or both, and had a control group with no intervention. Subjects were followed for an average period of 5.6 years. The incidence of diabetes was reduced in all three intervention groups and to an equal extent with 50 per cent reduction in the incidence of diabetes (Table 4.3). Some general points of interest emerged form this study.[15]

- Lifestyle interventions in the form of diet and physical activity for up to 6 years significantly reduced the development of diabetes.

- The effects of diet or exercise were similar, i.e. both reduced the risk of diabetes.

Table 4.3 The Da-Quing study from China

Intervention group	Cumulative incidence (%)
Control group	67
Diet only	44
Exercise only	41
Diet and exercise	46

- The risk of diabetes was reduced despite fairly modest reduction in body weight (approximately 2 kg).

- The increase in physical activity was modest but was sustained over the lifetime of the study.

- The effects were similar in obese and non-obese subjects.

The results of a recently published Diabetes Prevention Study (DPS) study from Finland have been extremely encouraging.[25] In this study the authors studied 522 subjects (172 men, 350 women). These were middle-aged subjects with a mean age of 55 and with a mean BMI of 31. Intervention in the control group consisted of verbal and written instructions about diet and exercise at baseline. The intervention group was given individualized dietary counselling aimed at reducing weight, total fat and saturated fat intake and increasing intake of fibre. This intervention was given in one-to-one sessions with the dietician seven times during the first year and 3 monthly thereafter. Physical activity counselling was also individually designed. It included both aerobic and resistance training, and increased walking with routine daily activities was encouraged. Some supervised activities were provided to train people. An oral glucose tolerance test (OGTT) was given annually on all subjects. If abnormal, diabetes was confirmed by a second OGTT test.

After an average follow-up of 3.2 years, subjects in the intervention group lost 4.2 kg of weight compared with 0.8 kg in the control group at year 1 with 3.5 and 0.8 kg at year 2, respectively. The cumulative incidence of diabetes in the intervention group was 11 per cent (95 per cent confidence interval, CI, 6–15) compared with 23 per cent (95 per cent CI 17–29) in the control group. Therefore, lifestyle intervention resulted in a total risk reduction of 58 per cent, results which were highly significant. Furthermore, the reduced incidence of diabetes was related to lifestyle changes. To interpret data in another way, 22 subjects with IGT will need to be treated for a year (or five subjects for 5 years) in this way to prevent one case of diabetes.

In the Diabetes Prevention Project (DPP) from the USA, 3234 subjects at high risk of type 2 diabetes were recruited. Eligibility criteria included age >25 years, minimal overweight and IGT as defined by WHO criteria. This study included 68 per cent women and 45 per cent of subjects were non-Caucasian (African-American, Hispanic, American Indians and Asian-Americans). The mean age was 51 years and BMI was 34 kgm^{-2}. Subjects were randomized to intensive lifestyle interventions ($n = 1979$), placebo ($n = 1082$) and metformin 850 mg twice daily ($n = 1073$). Intervention consisted of a goal of losing 7 per cent of weight and at least 150 min of exercise per week. The participants in the intensive exercise programme met case study managers on a one-to-one basis 16 times during the first 6 months and monthly thereafter. Primary outcome was diabetes based on results of an OGTT. The results of this study confirmed that type 2 diabetes could be prevented by lifestyle modifications and by pharmacological interventions. The risk of diabetes was reduced by both lifestyle changes in the form of diet and exercise and also by metformin treatment. After an average follow-up of 2.8 years, the incidence of diabetes was 11.0, 7.8, 4.8 cases per 100 person-years of follow-up in placebo, metformin and lifestyle interventions, respectively. The lifestyle intervention reduced diabetes incidence by 58 per cent and metformin by 38 per cent compared with placebo treatment.[26]

The findings of protective effect of lifestyle or metformin on diabetes were similar in men and women and in all racial groups. In general, lifestyle interventions were equally effective irrespective of age or Gender. They were more advantageous in older people with a lower body mass index, compared with younger persons and those with higher body mass index. Of major interest were the findings that both lifestyle intervention and metformin were similarly effective in restoring fasting glucose, but lifestyle intervention was more effective in restoring post-load glucose values.

In addition to these three landmark trials, other studies to prevent diabetes in populations at high risk but using pharmacological interventions are worth considering briefly. In The STOP-NIDDM study, acarbose was evaluated in a placebo-controlled trial in subjects with IGT.[27] After a mean follow-up of 3.3 years, the absolute risk reduction was 9 per cent in acarbose group and relative risk was reduced by 36 per cent when diabetes was confirmed with a second OGTT. In addition, in subjects with IGT there was a significant reversion to NGT.

In the TRIPOD study, 236 Hispanic women with gestational diabetes were randomized to troglitazone, which has now been withdrawn from the market. After a follow-up of 2.5 years, the incidence of diabetes was 12.3 and 5.4 per cent in control and intervention groups, giving a relative risk reduction of 56 per cent for future progression to diabetes.[28]

The results of the XENDOS trial have been published, in which orlistat and lifestyle intervention reduced risk of diabetes by 37 per cent compared with lifestyle alone. Another major consideration was that the orlistat group had a significant reduction in cardiovascular risk factors. These results underscore the fact that obesity prevention with whatever measures is needed to reduce diabetes and cardiovascular risk.[29] Other drugs, especially angiotensin-converting enzyme inhibitors (ACE-I), appear to be promising in preventing new-onset diabetes in a number of studies such as the HOPE and LIFE trials.[30,31] Studies are in progress (DREAM, NAVIGATOR) which will assess the impact of ramipril, rosiglitazone and the insulin scretagogue nateglinide on incident diabetes.[32,33]

The cost of interventions used in the DPS and DPP has been assessed in French, German and UK set-ups,[34] and was found to be higher for lifestyle interventions than for metformin. This should not come as a surprise, considering the huge cost of interventions which are needed for behaviour change so that one can adopt and maintain positive changes in lifestyle. Therefore, it might be argued that pharmacological interventions may appear to be a more attractive option for preventing diabetes. However, lifestyle interventions have the potential to impact multiple disease states. Diabetes prevention is a major public health issue in populations with high prevalence of type 2 diabetes, such as Asian Indians, as the rates of diabetes are projected to double over the next 20 years.[1] It remains for the health policy makers to make this a public health issue and urgent intervention trials are needed in these populations. The results of the Diabetes Prevention Trial in the Indian population are currently underway and we await the results with eagerness. However, lifestyle interventions in different racial groups may be particularly challenging,[17] suggesting that, when intervening with lifestyle measures, different strategies may need to be adopted in different racial groups. In a study reported from Tanzania in people of Hindu religion, simple dietary advice to eat less and exercise more in the form of walking for 30 min per day, resulted in protection from progression to diabetes.[35]

In most studies of lifestyle interventions, there was a tendency towards a reduction in risk factors for cardiovascular disease such as total and LDL-cholesterol and triglyceride and a decrease in systolic and diastolic blood pressure. There are few studies reported or in progress to date which will address the issue of whether treatment of IGT leads to prevention of cardiovascular disease. A high priority is not only to prevent or delay the onset of diabetes, but to reduce the future risk of macrovascular disease as well so that excess morbidity and mortality from manifestations of cardiovascular disease can be reduced. The STOP-NIDDM trial showed reversion to normal glucose tolerance in 30 per cent of subjects and a reduced risk of cardiovascular events. The long-term follow-up of DPP and DPS cohorts is awaited to see if interventions in these studies will result in reductions in long-term mortality from cardiovascular disease.

There would appear to be a greater urgency to develop strategies to prevent type 2 diabetes, given that diabetes seems to be appearing at a younger and younger age and in some countries in children and adolescents.[36] On the other hand, for the results of clinical trials to prevent diabetes to be meaningful, the results need to be generalizable, but the methods need to be affordable, practical and acceptable so that these can be easily implemented. It is quite clear that the intensity of intervention in the trials is not affordable even in the rich countries.[37]

In relation to the prevention of diabetes and coronary heart disease in the population at large, the following conclusions and recommendations may seem logical:

- Increase physical activity in the population at large by low-cost, low-key, but effective interventions (population approach).

- More intensive intervention should be aimed at those at high risk and a strategy is needed to identify these individuals (high risk approach).

- Those who are at high risk may need to be categorized in terms of their preference and ability to comply with various interventions so that intervention can be targeted. This may be crucial for the cost-effective utilization of resources, as some people may not choose to or be able to increase physical activity and therefore, may rely predominantly on dietary and/or pharmacological manipulations.

In a given population both approaches will be required to compliment each other, as interventions in high-risk people are more likely to be successful if all the population is geared to some sort of low-key interventions. However, this would need a clear and effective strategy to identify those at high risk by easy and effective means to target intervention.

References

1. King H, Aubert R, Herman W. Global burden of diabetes 1995–2025. Prevalence, numerical estimates, and projections. *Diabet Care* 1998; **21**: 1414–1431.
2. Greener M, Counting the cost of diabetes. *Costs Options Diabet* 1997; **10**: 4–5.
3. Knowler WC, Narayan KMV, Hanson RL, Nelson RG, Bennett PH, Tuommilehto J, Schersten B, Pettitt DJ. Perspective in diabetes. Preventing non-insulin-dependent diabetes. *Diabetes* 1995; **44**: 483–488.
4. Tuommilehto J, Knowler WC, Zimmet P. Primary prevention of non-insulin-dependent diabetes. *Diabetes/Metab Rev* 1992; **8**: 339–353.
5. Bennett PH. Impaired glucose tolerance – a target for intervention? *Arteriosclerosis* 1985; **5**: 315–317.
6. De Fronzo RA. Pathogenesis of type 2 (non-insulin dependant) diabetes mellitus: a balanced overview. *Diabetologia* 1992; **35**: 389–397.
7. Turner RC, Holman RR, Mathews DR, Peto J. Relative contributions of insulin deficiency and insulin resistance in maturity-onset diabetes. *Lancet* 1982; **i**: 596–598.
8. Gerich JE, Role of insulin resistance in the pathogenesis of type 2 (non-insulin dependant) diabetes mellitus. *Clin Endocrinol Metab* 1988; **2**: 307–326.
9. Nagi DK, Knowler WC, Charles MA, Lui QZ, Hanson RL, McCance DR, Pettitt DJ, Bennett PH. Early and late insulin response as predictors of NIDDM in Pima Indians with impaired glucose tolerance. *Diabetologia* 1995; **38**: 187–192.
10. Saad MF, Knowler WC, Pettitt DJ, Nelson RG, Mott DG, Bennett PH. The natural history of glucose intolerance in the Pima Indians. *New Engl J Med* 1988; **319**: 1500–1506.
11. Kadowaki T, Miyaki Y, Hagura R, Akanuma Y, Kuzuya N, Takaku F, Kosaka K. Risk factors for worsening to diabetes in subjects with impaired glucose tolerance. *Diabetologia* 1984; **26**: 44–49.
12. King H, Zimmet P, Raper LR, Balkau B. The natural history of impaired glucose tolerance in the micronesian population of Nauru: a 6 year follow-up study. *Diabetologia* 1984; **26**: 39–43.
13. World Health Organization. *Definition, Diagnosis and Classification of Diabetes Mellitus and its complications. Part 1: Diagnosis and classification of Diabetes Mellitus*. Report no. WHO/NCD/NCS/99.2. Geneva: Department of Non-Communicable Disease Surveillance, WHO, 1999.
14. Report of the Expert Committee on the Diagnosis and Classification of Diabetes Mellitus. *Diabetes Care* 1998; **21** (suppl. 1): S5–S19.

15. Pan X, Li G, Hu Y, Yang W, An Z, Hu Z, Lan J, Xiao J-Z, Cato H. Effects of diet and exercise in preventing NIDDM in people with impaired glucose tolerance. *Diabet Care* 1997; **20**: 537–544.

16. King H, Kriska AM. Prevention of type 2 diabetes by physical training. *Diabet Care* 1992; **15**: 1794–1799.

17. Narayan KMV, Hoskin M, Kozak D, Kriska A, Hanson RL, Pettitt DJ, Nagi DK, Bennett PH, Knowler WC. Randomised clinical trial of life style interventions in Pima Indians-a pilot study. *Diabet Med* 1998; **15**: 66–72.

18. Manson JE, Rimm RB, Stamfer MJ, Colditz GA, Willet WC, Krolewski AS, Rosner B, Hennekens CH, Speizer FE. A prospective study of exercise and incidence of diabetes among US male physicians. *JAMA* 1992; **268**: 63–67.

19. Helmrich SP, Ragland DR, Leung RW, Paffenbarger RS. Physical activity and reduced occupancy of non-insulin-dependent diabetes mellitus. *New Eng J Med* 1991; **325**: 147–152.

20. Manson JE, Rimm RB, Stamfer MJ, Colditz GA, Willet WC, Krolewski AS, Rosner B, Hennekens CH, Speizer FE. Physical activity and incidence of non-insulin-dependent diabetes in women. *Lancet* 1991; **338**: 774–778.

21. Burchfield CM, Sharp DS, Curb D, Rodriguez BL. Physical activity and incidence of diabetes: The Honolulu Heart Program. *Am J Epidemiol* 1995; **141**: 360–368.

22. Lynch J, Helmrich Sp, Lokka TA, Kaplan GA, Cohen RD, Salonen R, Salonen JT. Moderately intense physical activity and high levels of cardiorespiratory fitness reduce the risk of Non-insulin dependent diabetes mellitus in middle-aged men. *Arch Intern Med* 1996; **156**: 1307–1314.

23. Eriksson KF, Lindgarde F. No excess 12-year mortality in men with impaired glucose tolerance who participated in Malmo preventive trail with diet and exercise. *Diabetologia* 1998; **41**: 1010–1017.

24. Frisch RE, Wyshak G, Albright TE, Albright NL, Schiff I. Lower prevalence of diabetes in female former college athletes compared with non-athletes. *Diabetes* 1986; **35**: 1101–1105.

25. Tuomilehto J, Lindström J, Eriksson JG, Valle TT, Hämäläinen H, Ilanne-Parikka P, Keinänen-Kiukaanniemi S, Laakso M, Louheranta A, Rastas M, Salminen V, Uusitupa M. Prevention of type 2 diabetes mellitus by changes in lifestyle among subjects with impaired glucose tolerance. *New Engl J Med* 2001; **344**: 1343–1350.

26. The Diabetes Prevention Program Research Group. Reduction in the incidence of type 2 diabetes with lifestyle intervention or metformin. *New Engl J Med* 2002; **346**: 393–403.

27. Chiasson JL, Josse RG, Gomis R, Hanefield M, Karasik A, Laakso M, Acarbose for prevention of type 2 diabetes mellitus: the STOP-NIDDM randomised trial. *Lancet* 2002; **359**: 2072–2027.

28. Buchanan TA, Xiang AH, Peters RK, Kjos SL, Marroquin A, Goico J, Ochoa C, Tan S, Berkowitz K, Hodis HN, Azen SP. Preservation of pancreatic beta-cell function and prevention of type 2 diabetes by pharmacological treatment of insulin resistance in high-risk Hispanic women. *Diabetes* 2002; **51**: 2796–2803.

29. Torgerson JS, Boldrin MN, Hauptman J, Sjorstrom L. Xenical in the prevention of diabetes in obese subjects (XENDOS) study. A randomised study of Orlistat as an adjunct to lifestyle changes for the prevention of type 2 diabetes in obese patients. *Diabet Care* 2004; **27**: 155–161.

30. Heart Outcomes Prevention Evaluation (HOPE) Study. Effects of ramipril on cardiovascular and microvascular outcomes in people with diabetes mellitus: results of the HOPE study and MICRO-HOPE substudy. *Lancet* 2000; **355**: 253–259.

31. Lindholm LH, Ibsen H, Daholf B, Deverux RB, Beevers G, de Faire U, Fyhrquist F, Julius S, Kjeldon SE, Kristianson K. Cardiovascular morbidity and mortality in patients with diabetes

in the Lorsartan Intervention For Endpoint reduction in hypertension study (LIFE): a randomised trial against Atenolol. *Lancet* 2003; **359**: 1004–1010.

32. Rationale, design and recruitment of a large, simple intervention trial of diabetes prevention. The DREAM trial. *Diabetologia* 2004; **47**: 1519–1527.

33. Simpson RW, Shaw JE, Zimmet PZ. The prevention of type 2 diabetes – lifestyle changes or pharmacotherapy? A challenge for 21st century. *Diabet Res Clin Pract* 2003; **59**: 165–180.

34. Palmer AJ, Roze S, Valentine-William J, Spinas GA, Shaw JE, Zimmet P. Intensive life style changes or metformin in patients with impaired glucose tolerance: modelling the long-term implications of the diabetes prevention programme in Australia, France, Germany, Switzerland and the United Kingdom. *Clin Ther* 2004; **26**: 304–321.

35. Ramaya KL, Swai ABM, Alberti KGMM, McLarty D. Lifestyle changes decrease rates of glucose intolerance and cardiovascular (CVD) risk factors: a six-year intervention study in a high risk Hindu Indian sub-community. *Diabetologia* 1992; **35** (suppl. 1): A60.

36. Dean H, Flett B. Natural history of Type 2 diabetes diagnosed in childhood: long term follow up in young adult years. *Diabetologia* 2002; **51**: A24.

37. Zimmet P, Shaw J, Alberti KGMM. Preventing type 2 diabetes and the Dysmetabolic syndrome in the real world: a realistic view. *Diabet Med* 2003; **20**: 693–702.

5

Exercise, Metabolic Syndrome and Type 2 Diabetes

Dinesh Nagi

5.1 Physical Activity in Type 2 Diabetes

The importance of regular physical activity in the management of diabetes has been realized for centuries[1] and regular physical activity has been advocated to have an important role in the management of type 2 diabetes.[2,3] Physical activity when used in conjunction with diet was the sole form of treatment for diabetes in the pre-insulin era. Over the last two decades the potential benefits of physical activity in type 2 diabetes have become clearer. The mechanisms by which regular physical activity may confer these benefits are becoming better understood.[4] The role of physical activity in the prevention of type 2 diabetes[5,6] is discussed in Chapter 4.

Physical activity is an important component of the treatment plan for diabetes due to its effects on plasma glucose concentrations and other associated risk factors. Therefore, to fully realize the importance of regular physical activity in the management of type 2 diabetes, the beneficial effects on other risk factors for cardiovascular disease, such as obesity, hypertension, hyperlipidaemia and abnormalities of fibrinolysis/coagulation, which are an integral part of the 'metabolic syndrome', must be taken into account. Although hyperglycaemia is causally related to the microvascular complications of diabetes, the association between hyperglycaemia and macrovascular disease is less clear.[7] No randomized trials of any treatment modalities in type 2 diabetes have shown that good glycaemic control reduces mortality from macrovascular disease, which is a major cause of mortality in these subjects.[8] In real life, many patients with type 2 diabetes are

Exercise and Sport in Diabetes, 2nd Edition   Edited by Dinesh Nagi
© 2005 John Wiley & Sons, Ltd.

sedentary and unable to increase their physical activity levels. There are several reasons for this, but it is partly due to chronic complications of diabetes or associated medical conditions.[9,10] Despite potential benefits, which I will discuss later, the uptake of regular physical activity in patients with type 2 diabetes remains poor and improving this represents a major challenge for behaviour therapists and clinicians.

The purpose of this article is to review the relevant literature so as to critically appraise the role of physical activity in our current approach to diabetes management. There are no long-term studies on the impact of physical activity on glycaemic control and on complications of type 2 diabetes. Most of the data are from studies with short follow-up and inadequate randomization.

As we routinely recommend physical activity as an essential part of the management strategy for patients with type 2 diabetes, answers to the following fundamental questions need to be explored.

1. Does it have short- and long-term effects on glycaemic control?

2. Does it have a beneficial effect on other associated risk factors such as hypertension and dyslipidaemia?

3. Does it improve the quality of life in diabetics?

4. Does it have any effect on the natural history of cardiovascular disease?

5. Does it reduce the long-term mortality?

6. Are there any effects on specific complications of diabetes?

Having explored these, we will be in a position to assess the risk–benefit ratio of physical activity in order to better understand the reasons for using it as an integral part of the treatment plan for type 2 diabetes mellitus (see Chapter 6).

If we come to the conclusion that exercise is potentially beneficial, we will need to address the best methods to improve uptake and compliance with physical activity. We will also need to consider what role we as health professionals play in promoting physical activity and supporting those who are contemplating being active or are already engaged in physical activity (see Chapter 12).

5.2   Type 2 Diabetes, Insulin Resistance and the Metabolic Syndrome

It is now generally agreed that type 2 diabetes results from a combination of insulin resistance and β-cell dysfunction.[11] However, type 2 diabetes is a heterogeneous disorder and the relative role of these two in the pathogenesis of type 2 diabetes may vary in different populations and also among subjects within the same population.[12] There is evidence that insulin deficiency and autoimmunity may play a relatively greater role in a small proportion of Caucasian subjects.[13,14] The natural history of the disease suggests that increasing duration of diabetes and worsening of hyperglycaemia eventually lead to a state of marked β-cell failure.[15] Therefore, a substantial proportion of subjects with type 2 diabetes will eventually need insulin treatment to achieve good glycaemic control and improved quality of life, if not for immediate survival.[16]

During the early twentieth century, Himsworth showed that subjects with diabetes can be broadly categorized into those who are 'insulin sensitive' (now known at type 1) and 'insulin insensitive' (now known as type 2) based on their plasma glucose responses to an oral glucose load given together with subcutaneous insulin injection.[17] Subsequently, using sophisticated techniques, it has been shown that insulin resistance is a universal feature of type 2 diabetes.[18] Interestingly, up to 25 per cent of non-diabetic individuals may also have insulin resistance which is quantitatively similar to what is seen in subjects with type 2 diabetes.[19]

Studies done during the early 1960s found that insulin resistance, hyperinsulinaemia and impaired glucose tolerance were frequently associated with coronary artery disease.[20,21] In 1984, Modan et al. showed an association between hypertension, glucose intolerance, obesity and hyperinsulinaemia. She proposed that insulin resistance and its consequent hyperinsulinaemia may be a common pathophysiologic basis for this interesting association.[22] Reaven popularized the existence of multiple metabolic risk factors that seem to cluster in certain individuals, which he called 'syndrome X'. This syndrome is characterized by glucose intolerance, hyperinsulinaemia, increased serum triglyceride, decreased high-density lipoprotein (HDL) cholesterol and the presence of hypertension.[23] Reaven proposed that insulin resistance and consequent hyperinsulinaemia were the common antecedents for this metabolic syndrome (Figure 5.1) and that this syndrome may be involved in the aetiology and clinical course of type 2 diabetes, hypertension and coronary artery disease. Since then other variables such as plasminogen activator inhibitor (PAI-1) and fibrinogen have been added to the ever growing components of this syndrome, which is now more commonly known as 'the metabolic syndrome'.[24] A majority of subjects who have features of the metabolic syndrome are obese but also have a central distribution of fat (increased waist-to-hip ratio), which is more strongly associated with insulin resistance and hyperinsulinaemia.[25] Physical inactivity is suggested to be an important factor leading to the development of this metabolic syndrome.[26]

The relationship of insulin resistance, hyperinsulinaemia, and central obesity with adverse cardiovascular risk factors clearly exists, as shown in various studies,[27,28] despite poorly understood mechanisms.[29,30] There is still considerable debate as to wheather it is insulin resistance or its consequent hyperinsulinaemia which is the proximate cause of the metabolic syndrome, although epidemiological

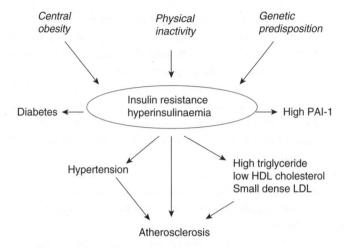

Figure 5.1   Components of the metabolic syndrome

data would be against high insulin levels being responsible for the metabolic syndrome.[26]

It is now agreed that clustering of multiple risk factors in subjects with diabetes may predate clinical diagnosis of diabetes by many years and contributes to the excess risk of cardiovascular disease in these subjects before and around the time of diagnosis of type 2 diabetes and thereafter.[31] Data from the San Antonio Heart Study showed higher levels of cardiovascular risk factors and hyperinsulinaemia at baseline in subjects who developed diabetes during the 8 year follow-up compared with those who did not. Findings of the MRFIT trial showed that, in subjects with type 2 diabetes, the risk of cardiovascular death increased sharply in those who had two or more risk factors,[32] confirming an earlier well-known finding of increased cardiovascular mortality in subjects with diabetes observed in the Framingham data.

In subjects with type 2 diabetes, physical inactivity is related both to obesity and to a central or abdominal distribution of fat.[33] Lack of regular physical activity may also contribute to the development of insulin resistance either directly or through weight gain, so that an increase in physical activity might be expected to improve the metabolic syndrome associated with insulin resistance in subjects with type 2 diabetes.

5.3   Effect of Exercise on the Metabolic Syndrome of Type 2 Diabetes

Work by O'Dea with Australian aborigines showed that reverting to a traditional lifestyle of hunting and gathering was associated with a marked improvement in glucose intolerance and a reduction in plasma triglyceride and blood pressure.[34] On average, fasting plasma glucose fell by $5 \, \text{mmol} \, \text{l}^{-1}$ and subjects lost $10 \, \text{kg}$ in weight over a 7 week period. These changes in weight and plasma glucose were not solely due to increase in physical activity, as their diet changed both in quality and quantity. Nevertheless, this study provided evidence that lifestyle modifications with changes in physical activity and diet can cause significant weight loss and probably improve the various components of the metabolic syndrome.

Furthermore, Rogers *et al.*[35] showed that the effects of exercise on insulin resistance and plasma glucose, become apparent after a fairly short period of time and without any weight loss. In this study, a 7 day programme of moderate intensity exercise, without any changes in body weight, was associated with improved glucose tolerance and a fall in prandial insulin concentrations in subjects with type 2 diabetes. In addition to a fall in fasting and post-prandial insulin levels after exercise, there was a tendency toward an earlier insulin peak, suggesting that exercise has the potential to modify both insulin resistance and insulin secretion, two of the fundamental defects implicated in the pathogenesis of type 2 diabetes.

A study by Wing *et al.*[36] confirmed the possible contribution to the benefits of exercise alone or when exercise is combined with diet. In this study subjects with type 2 diabetes were randomized to a programme of diet alone or diet and exercise. All subjects were given similar dietary advice and subjects in the exercise group in addition walked 3 miles a day three to four times per week. Subjects were assessed over a 60 week period. In this study, the diet and exercise group on average lost twice the amount of weight over an initial 20 week period, but were also able to maintain this difference at 60 weeks compared with those randomized to diet alone (Figure 5.2). In this study, glycaemic control improved to a similar extent in both groups. Further analyses of subjects showed that, in the whole group (data combined for diet and diet + exercise groups), the magnitude of improvement

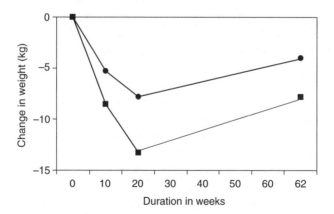

Figure 5.2 Effect of diet alone or diet + exercise on weight loss in subjects with type 2 diabetes. Adapted from Wing *et al.*[36]

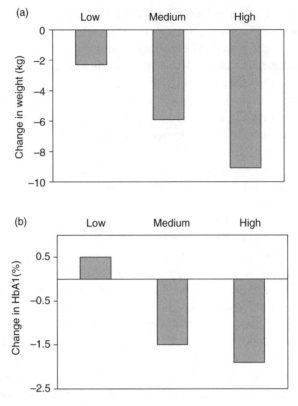

Figure 5.3 Changes in weight (a) and glycated haemoglobin (b) by physical activity level in subjects with type 2 diabetes. Adapted from Wing *et al.*[36]

in glycaemic control as judged by HbA1 and the degree of weight loss were more marked in those who were more physically active [Figure 5.3 (a,b)]. In addition, a higher proportion of subjects in diet and exercise group (83 per cent) were able to reduce their drug treatment for diabetes compared with the diet alone group (37 per cent). Although this study had a small number of subjects, the results were extremely encouraging to show that exercise when combined with diet can lead to more weight loss and help to maintain weight compared with diet alone.

A study of community-based intervention from New Mexico showed similar benefits but over a longer time period.[37] In this study, subjects who took part in the intervention lost an average 4 kg in weight, lowered fasting plasma glucose by 2.5 mmol l^{-1}, and up to 20 per cent of the subjects were able to discontinue their hypoglycaemic medication. However, the study was non-randomized and participation in the programme was voluntary. The uptake rates of such a programme were not given and such community-based interventions, although attractive in principle, seem to suffer from problems of long-term compliance, difficulties in organization and delivery of effective intervention.

A randomized study by Vanninen et al.[38] analysing the impact of physical fitness on glycaemic control showed significant initial decreases in body weight, fasting blood glucose and HbA1c. They observed that physical fitness as assessed by VO_{2max}, was lower in subjects with type 2 diabetes. There was an inverse correlation between VO_{2max} and HbA1c, suggesting that improvement in physical fitness may be associated with better glycaemic control. However, over a longer time period improvement was only observed in female subjects, although with some fall in blood glucose and insulin levels at one year in most subjects.

Larsen et al.[39] analysed the effects of moderate exercise on post-prandial glucose homeostasis. They showed a beneficial effect of exercise on glycaemia and insulin levels but the effect persisted only in the post-absorptive phase of that meal and not the following meal. They also found that a reduction in the caloric content of the meal, equivalent to what was spent during exercise, had the same effect. The practical implications are that a patient with diabetes could choose to eat ad-libitum and subsequently expend these calories by exercise. While this approach may be useful for lean subjects, it would hardly be of practical value in obese subjects with type 2 diabetes where weight reduction is the main aim and some sort of caloric restriction is almost always essential.

Lehmann et al.[40] showed that a regular aerobic exercise programme at 50–70 per cent maximal effort for 3 months led to a 20 per cent reduction in fasting plasma triglyceride concentrations and an increase in HDL lipoprotein subfraction. In this study, there was a significant reduction in systolic and diastolic blood pressure and more importantly a significant fall in waist-to-hip ratio, suggesting a predominant loss of abdominal fat. These effects were independent of body weight and glycaemic control. There were no significant changes in the glycaemic control in the intervention group, although in the control group HbA1c rose by 0.6 per cent. All these studies showed clear-cut benefits, but were short-term studies.

There have been a number of studies published on the effects of exercise in type 2 diabetes; their findings are somewhat varied and most studies were of short duration. There have been no studies of adequate statistical power to guide us on the glycaemic effects of exercise. HbA1c was reduced in some and not in others, therefore it may be useful to look at the meta-analyses of studies of exercise and glycaemic control. Boule et al.[41] examined the effects of exercise on glycaemic control and body weight and concluded that exercise reduces Hba1c by approximately 0.66 per cent, an amount which may be clinically significant in the long run. They did not find any greater weight loss in the exercise group. They found that the differences in HbA1c between the exercise and the control group were not mediated by differences in weight, exercise intensity and the amount of exercise. They concluded that exercise does not have to reduce weight to have a beneficial effect on glucose control.

Barnard et al.[42] also showed that the effect of exercise on fasting plasma glucose was related to pharmacological treatment of diabetes and was larger in those on diet alone compared with those on oral hypoglycaemic or insulin treatment. This observation would suggest that exercise is likely to be beneficial in those who are early in the natural history of disease progression of type 2 diabetes.

5.4   What Kind of Exercise, Aerobic or Resistance Training?

There has always been controversy about what kind of exercise is likely to be beneficial in patients with type 2 diabetes. However, recent studies have shown that aerobic exercise alone, or combined with resistance or strength training, is likely to be beneficial in improving metabolic control in subjects with type 2 diabetes.[43–45]

In a widely publicized study by Eriksson and Lindgarde it was clear that an outpatient exercise programme can be maintained successfully for up to 6 years. This was a non-randomized study of primary prevention of type 2 diabetes, which also included 41 patients with known type 2 diabetes and 161 subjects with impaired glucose tolerance (IGT). There was a significant improvement in glucose tolerance and post-prandial insulin concentrations despite fairly modest amount of weight loss.[46] In 28 per cent of subjects with diabetes, the glucose tolerance had returned to normal, 26 per cent of subjects reverted to IGT and 46 per cent were still classified as diabetic. In subjects who had IGT at baseline, 69 per cent had normal glucose tolerance and 21 per cent still had IGT; 11 per cent had developed diabetes compared with 21 per cent in the control group. The most valid and encouraging conclusion of this study was the demonstration that the outpatient-based exercise programme was successfully maintained for up to 5 years.

Overall, exercise and physical activity is considered to have a moderate effect on glycaemic control. This is due to the lack of long-term data and sustainability of the effect in a condition which is progressive in nature, and different pharmacological interventions are generally required with increasing disease duration.

5.5   Effects on Cardiovascular Risk Factors

Most of the studies discussed above have also shown beneficial effects on lipids and blood pressure. The study by Rogers et al.[35] showed a fall in systolic blood pressure of 6 mmHg and a 33 per cent reduction in plasma triglyceride concentrations. Wing et al.[36] showed a significant reduction in serum cholesterol and plasma triglyceride concentrations which was significant at 10 weeks but not at one year. HDL cholesterol levels remained higher after a one year follow-up, but no changes were observed in systolic and diastolic blood pressures. Schneider et al.[47] in their study showed improvements of approximately 25 per cent in plasma triglyceride but no change in LDL cholesterol. Similar beneficial effects were maintained in the Malmo study for up to 6 years. Krotkiewsky et al.[48] noticed that the best response occurred in subjects who had highest baseline fasting insulin concentrations, a finding also confirmed by Schneider et al.[47] These findings would suggest that the mechanisms for changes in lipids following exercise are intimately related to changes in insulin resistance.

Increase in physical activity is associated with a fall in plasma triglyceride and a rise in HDL cholesterol.[49,50] The effect on LDL cholesterol is only modest, but there may be beneficial effects on LDL composition. It would also appear that to gain the maximum benefits in terms of improvements in lipids, moderate intensity exercise may be required. For instance, in non-diabetic subjects, the effects on lipids increased with increasing exercise in a dose-dependent manner up to a distance of 40 miles per week.[51]

Insulin resistance is universally associated with high plasma triglyceride and low HDL cholesterol concentrations.[52] Impaired LPL activity is usually associated with insulin-resistant states and exercise is likely to achieve beneficial effects on plasma triglyceride and HDL cholesterol by influencing both muscle and hepatic lipoprotein lipase activity.[49] The former change will lead to a greater extraction and clearance of very-low-density lipoprotein (VLDL) at the periphery and the latter to less release of VLDL into circulation from the liver. In addition other possible mechanisms such as enhanced reverse cholesterol transport may be important. Some of the effects of exercise on lipids may be indirect and related to loss of abdominal fat. As a consequence, there is less mobilization of free fatty acids (FFA) from abdominal fat to liver, thereby reducing hepatic VLDL production.[53]

Essential hypertension has been intimately linked to insulin resistance.[54] One mechanism by which hyperinsulinaemia is related to blood pressure in type 2 diabetes is through its effects on the sympathetic nervous system and renal sodium handling.[55,56] A reduction in blood pressure following intervention with an increase in physical activity is significantly related to improvement in insulin sensitivity and correlated with reduced fasting hyperinsulinaemia and independent of change in weight.[57] Regular physical activity may lower blood pressure, on average, by 8–10 mmHg. Improvement in blood pressure of this magnitude, if sustained, has the potential to significantly modify cardiovascular risk in type 2 diabetes.

There are data to suggest that regular physical activity may have a beneficial effect on fibrinolysis, although the effects remain somewhat inconsistent. Schneider et al.[58] showed improved fibrinolysis following 6 weeks of exercise in subjects with type 2 diabetes. Gris et al.[54] showed similar benefits and these were associated with lower levels of PAI-1. PAI-1 has been shown to be related to insulin resistance. The lowering of PAI-1 and fibrinolysis is also related to improvements in circulating insulin and plasma triglyceride concentrations, both of which are related to insulin resistance.[60] There are no long-term studies on the effects of exercise on fibrinolysis. As raised levels of PAI-1 are shown to predict recurrence of acute myocardial infarction in non-diabetic and diabetic subjects,[61,62] it is possible that the effects of exercise in lowering PAI-1 and plasma fibrinogen levels may produce long-term reduction in cardiovascular events. In addition, combined aerobic and resistance training has been shown to be beneficial for endothelial dysfunction, which contributes to the macrovascular disease so frequently seen in patients with type 2 diabetes.[63]

However, the overall compliance with outpatient-based exercise programmes remains poor.[9,10] In a study by Schneider *et al.*, compliance dropped to 20 per cent by the end of 12 months. As in the above studies, subjects who took part in this programme of diet and exercise showed significant weight loss and lower fasting plasma glucose and lower fasting plasma triglyceride levels at 3 months, which were maintained for up to one year. Several key observations in this study are worth reviewing. Firstly, the best predictors of long-term compliance were self-referral, participation from spouse and female sex. Secondly, even those subjects who dropped out of the programme at 3 months were still taking part in some sort of physical activity when interviewed a year later. In the study by Wing *et al.*[36] compliance to exercise as judged by calories expended was excellent for the duration of the study, even though after 20 weeks subjects were left to do their walking by themselves. Therefore is seems that an initial intensive training period may be essential to long-term compliance. Therefore, formalized programmes may best be used for initial patient education to prepare individuals to exercise safely and appropriately on their own, choosing activities which they enjoy and which fit into their daily lifestyle.

5.6   Regulation of Carbohydrate Metabolism During Exercise in Type 2 Diabetes

The effects of exercise on carbohydrate metabolism are discussed in detail in Chapter 1. In non-diabetic subjects during exercise, there is a strong negative relationship between plasma glucose concentration and hepatic glucose production. However, the regulation of carbohydrate (CHO) metabolism during and immediately after exercise differs in subjects with type 2 diabetes compared with those without. Hepatic glucose production during exercise is generally reduced in type 2 diabetes and the strong negative relationship between plasma glucose and hepatic glucose output, as seen in non-diabetic subjects, is generally lacking. This would suggest that the feedback control of glucose production from the liver by plasma glucose is impaired in diabetes.[64] A study by Kjaer *et al.*[65] showed that, 10 min after an acute bout of exercise, there was a rise in plasma glucose which was of higher magnitude in subjects with type 2 diabetes due to excess hepatic glucose production. Furthermore, this initial rise in plasma glucose due to exaggerated counter-regulatory hormone responses was followed by a period during which insulin sensitivity seemed to continue to improve for up to a 24 h period. A study by Schneider *et al.*[66] showed that, after 6 weeks of physical training, there was a blunting of exercise-induced increase in the counter-regulatory response in non-diabetic but not in subjects with diabetes. Exercise resulted in a decrease in plasma glucose in subjects with diabetes but an increase in non-diabetic subjects 30 min after exercise.

From these studies, it is clear that, in subjects with type 2 diabetes, because of exaggerated counter-regulatory responses, maximum dynamic exercise results in a short period of hyperglycaemia. However, this is followed by a period of 'insulin sensitization' with a beneficial effect on glucose utilization. In summary, glucose turnover after exercise in type 2 diabetes is heterogeneous and may show a fall or a sustained rise or no change. These differences are likely to be due to impaired non-pancreatic hormonal responses,[65,66] but also the heterogeneity of type 2 diabetes mellitus, as well as the contribution by insulin resistance and insulin secretion.

5.7   Effect of Physical Activity on Insulin Sensitivity

The earliest indication that exercise has the potential to improve insulin sensitivity was put forward by Bjorntorp.[67] After 12 weeks of exercise or physical training, there was a substantial fall in circulating fasting and post-prandial insulin concentrations without any changes in plasma glucose levels.[68] Subsequently, Rosenthal et al.[69] showed that insulin sensitivity was directly related to physical training as measured by VO_{2max}, both in men and women. Studies using a hyperinsulinaemic clamp showed that insulin stimulated glucose uptake increased following a single bout of physical training.[64,70] This improvement in insulin sensitivity was localized to exercising muscles as a way of replenishing glycogen stores depleted during exercise, while non-exercising muscles were relatively insulin-resistant immediately following exercise.[71,72]

The mechanism of glucose disposal may differ in subjects with type 2 diabetes who are treated with dietary modification alone compared with those treated with diet and exercise.[73] In this study, subjects who exercised in addition to diet mainly used non-oxidative (glycogen synthesis) route for glucose disposal while those on diet alone did so by oxidative pathways (glucose oxidation). These observations also provide a pathophysiologic basis for an additive effect of diet and exercise on insulin sensitivity. Devlin et al.[70] showed similar results in subjects with type 2 diabetes (i.e. the effect of exercise was on non-oxidative glucose disposal). After a single bout of exercise in subjects with type 2 diabetes, both peripheral and hepatic insulin sensitivity improved (Figure 5.4). They also found lower basal hepatic glucose output after exercise which was accompanied by lower fasting plasma glucose the morning after exercise.[70]

There is still no universal agreement as to the intensity and duration of exercise needed to improve insulin sensitivity. Most studies suggest that exercise intensity of at least 40–50 per cent VO_{2max} (which is considered to be of moderate intensity) is needed to improve insulin sensitivity.[74] Exercise of this intensity is associated with some glycogen depletion, which may be a prerequisite for enhancing glucose disposal following exercise.[70] The underlying cellular mechanisms by which these

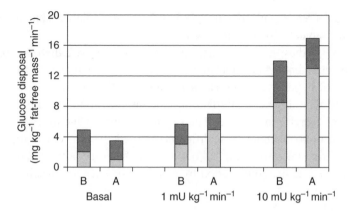

Figure 5.4 Effect of exercise on oxidative (OGD) and non-oxidative glucose disposal (NODG) at baseline and during low dose ($1\,mU\,kg^{-1}\,min^{-1}$) and high dose ($10\,mU\,kg^{-1}\,min^{-1}$) hyperinsulinaemic euglycaemic clamp studies in subjects with type 2 diabetes. B = before exercise; A = after exercise. Reproduced from Devlin *et al.*[71]

beneficial effects occur are not fully elucidated. Studies have shown that exercise improves insulin receptor numbers[75] as well as tissue levels of glucose transporters (GLUT 4), thereby facilitating glucose transport into the cells, and its disposal through insulin-sensitive pathways.[76]

Recently published studies have examined the impact of exercise on cellular mechanisms involved with non-insulin stimulated glucose uptake following exercise. Musi *et al.*[77] showed that $\alpha2$ AMP-activated protein kinase increases after exercise in type 2 diabetes.[77] The expression of other isoforms remained normal. They suggested that this mechanism may play an important role in the non-insulin-mediated glucose uptake after a bout of exercise.

The improvement in insulin sensitivity following a single episode of exercise has been shown to last for up to 60 h, and is completely normalized to pre-exercise levels by 3–5 days.[78] Repeated bouts of moderate intensity exercise may, however, provide adaptive mechanisms which are associated with a long-term increase in insulin sensitivity.[79,80] From a practical point, it seems likely that modest fall in plasma glucose levels following repeated bouts of physical activity at intervals not longer than 48–60 h may be associated with long-term changes in glycaemia control.

Although type 2 diabetes is an insulin-resistant state, both at periphery and at hepatic level, glucose utilization during exercise is probably higher compared with non-diabetic subjects due to mechanisms discussed above. It is also quite clear this is an acute effect of exercise and therefore exercise has to be taken on a regular basis to enhance insulin sensitivity. Since skeletal muscle is the major site of glucose uptake, large muscle groups need to be exercised, a view supported by the fact that one leg exercised alone does not enhance total body insulin sensitivity.[81]

To summarize, regular physical activity in subjects with type 2 diabetes is associated with improved short- and probably long-term glycaemic control.

Regular physical activity when combined with dietary modification leads to more profound weight loss and may also help in long-term weight maintenance. Weight loss is a necessary prerequisite for accruing the benefits on glycaemic control due to exercise. In addition, there are beneficial changes in associated cardiovascular risk factors such as blood pressure, dyslipidaemia and abnormalities of thrombosis and coagulation. The benefits of exercise on glycaemia would appear to be most marked around the time of diagnosis and early in the natural history of disease progression. These changes appear to be intimately related to beneficial changes in insulin sensitivity.

References

1. Sushruta SCS. *Vaidya Jadavaji Trikamji Acharia*, 13th revision, 3rd ed. Bombay: Nirnyar Sagar Press, 1938 (original book published in 500 BC).
2. American Diabetes Association. Exercise and NIDDM (technical review). *Diabetes Care* 1990; **13**: 785–789.
3. American Diabetes Association. Diabetes mellitus and exercise (position statement). *Diabetes Care* 1990; **13**: 804–805.
4. Schneider SH, Morgado A. Effects of fitness and physical training on carbohydrate metabolism and associated cardiovascular risk factors in patients with diabetes. *Diabet Rev* 1995; **3**: 378–407.
5. Knowler WC, Narayan KMV, Hanson RL, Nelson RG, Bennett PH, Tuommilehto J, Schersten B, Pettitt DJ. Perspective in diabetes. Preventing non-insulin-dependent diabetes. *Diabetes* 1995; **44**: 483–488.
6. National Institutes of Health. Non-insulin Dependent Diabetes Primary Prevention Trial. *NIH Guide Grants Cont* 1993; **22**: 1–20.
7. Barrett-Connor E. Does hyperglycaemia really causes coronary artery disease? *Diabetes Care* 1997; **20**: 1620–1623.
8. Panzram G. Mortality and survival in type 2 (non-insulin-dependent) diabetes mellitus. *Diabetologia* 1987; **30**: 123–131.
9. Samaras K, Ashwell S, Mackintosh A-M, Campbell LV, Chisholm DJ. Exercise in NIDDM: are we missing the point? *Diab Med* 1996; **13**: 780–781.
10. Schneider SH, Khanchadurian AK, Amorosa LF, Clemow L, Ruderman NB. Ten-year experience with an exercise-based outpatient life-style modification program in the treatment of diabetes mellitus. *Diabetes Care* 1992; **15** (suppl. 4): 1800–1810.
11. DeFronzo RA. Pathogenesis of type 2 (non-insulin-dependent) diabetes mellitus: a balanced overview. *Diabetologia* 1992; **35**: 389–397.
12. Turner RC, Holman RR, Matthews DR, Peto J. Relative contributions of insulin deficiency and insulin resistance in maturity-onset diabetes. *Lancet* 1982; **i**: 596–598.
13. Temple RC, Carrington CA, Luzio SD, Owens DR, Schneider AE, Sobey WJ, Halesÿ CN. Insulin deficiency in non-insulin-dependent diabetes. *Lancet* 1989; **i**: 293–295.
14. Groop L, Miettinen A, Groop PH, Meri S, Koskimies S, Bottazzo GF. Organ-specific autoimmunity and HLA-DR antigen as markers for b-cell destruction in patients with type II diabetes. *Diabetes* 1988; **37**: 99–103.
15. DeFronzo RA. The triumvirate: β-cell, muscle, liver – a collusion responsible for NIDDM. *Diabetes* 1988; **37**: 667–687.

16. DeFronzo RA, Ferrannini E, Koivisto V. New concepts in the pathogenesis and treatment of non-insulin dependent diabetes mellitus. *Am J Med* 1983; **74**: 52–81.

17. Himsworth H. Diabetes mellitus: a differentiation into insulin sensitive and insulin insensitive types. *Lancet* 1936; **i**: 127–130.

18. Gerich JE. Role of insulin resistance in the pathogenesis of type 2 (non-insulin-dependent) diabetes mellitus. *Clin Endocrinol Metab* 1988; **2**: 307–326.

19. Hollenbeck C, Reaven GM. Variations in insulin-stimulated glucose uptake in healthy individuals with normal glucose tolerance. *J Clin Endocrinol Metab* 1987; **64**: 1169–1173.

20. Welborn TA, Breckenridge A, Rubinstein AH, Dollery CT, Fraser TR. Serum insulin in essential hypertension and peripheral vascular disease. *Lancet* 1969; **i**: 1078–1080.

21. Nikkila EA, Miettinen TA, Vesene M-R, Pelkonen R. Plasma insulin in coronary artery disease. *Lancet* 1965; **ii**: 508–511.

22. Modan M, Halkin H, Almog S, Lusky A, Eshkol A, Shefi M, Shitrit A and Fuchs Z. Hyperinsulinemia: a link between hypertension, obesity and glucose intolerance. *J Clin Invest* 1985; **75**: 809–817.

23. Reaven GM. Role of insulin resistance in human disease. *Diabetes* 1988; **37**: 1595–1607.

24. Landin K, Tenghorn L, Smith U. Elevated fibrinogen and plasminogen activator inhibitor (PAI-1) in hypertension are related to metabolic risk factors for cardiovascular disease. *J Intern Med* 1990; **227**: 273–278.

25. Pouliot M-C, Despres J-P, Nadeau A, Moorjani S, Prud-Homme D, Lupien PJ, Tremblay A, Bouchard C. Visceral obesity in man. Associations with glucose tolerance, plasma insulin, and lipoprotein levels. *Diabetes* 1992; **41**: 826–834.

26. Zimmet PZ. Hyperinsulinemia, how innocent a bystander? *Diabetes Care* 1993; **16**: 56–70.

27. DeFronzo RA, Ferrannini E. Insulin resistance: a multifaceted syndrome responsible for NIDDM, obesity, hypertension, dyslipidaemia and atherosclerotic vascular disease. *Diabetes Care* 1991; **14**: 173–194.

28. Haffner SM, Valdez RA, Hazuda HP, Mitchell BD, Morales PA, Stern MP. Prospective analysis of the insulin resistance syndrome (syndrome X). *Diabetes* 1992; **41**: 715–722.

29. Stern MP. Diabetes and cardiovascular disease: the 'common soil' hypothesis. *Diabetes* 1995; **44**: 369–374.

30. Kissebah AH, Vydelingum N, Murray R, Evans DJ, Hartz AJ, Kalkhoff RK, Adams PW. Relation of body fat distribution to metabolic complications of obesity. *J Clin Endocrinol Metab* 1982; **54**: 254–260.

31. Haffner SM, Stern MP, Hazuda HP, Mitchell BD, Patterson JK. Cardiovascular risk factors in confirmed prediabetic individuals. Does the clock for coronary heart disease start ticking before the onset of clinical diabetes? *JAMA* 1990; **263**: 2893–2898.

32. Stamler J, Vaccaro O, Neaton JD, Wentworth D. Diabetes, Other risk factors, mortality for men screened in the Multiple Risk Factor Intervention Trial. *Diabetes Care* 1993; **16**: 434–444.

33. Kriska AM, LaPorte RE. The association of physical activity with obesity, fat distribution and glucose intolerance in Pima Indians. *Diabetologia* 1993; **36**: 863–869.

34. O'Dea K. Marked improvement in carbohydrate and lipid metabolism in diabetes Australian Aborigines after temporary reversion to a traditional lifestyle. *Diabetes* 1984; **33**: 596–603.

35. Rogers MA, Yamamoto C, King DS, Hagberg JM, Ehasani AA, Holloszy JO. Improvement in glucose tolerance after 1 week of exercise in patients with mild NIDDM. *Diabetes Care* 1988; **11**: 613–618.

36. Wing RR, Epstein LH, Paternostro-Bayles M, Kriska A, Nowalk MP, Gooding W. Exercise in a behavioral weight control programme for obese patients with type II diabetes. *Diabetologia* 1988; **31**: 902–909.

37. Heath GW, Leonard BE, Wilson RH, Kendrick JS, Powell KE. Community-based exercise intervention: Zuni diabetes project. *Diabetes Care* 1987; **10**: 579–583.

38. Vanninen E, Uusitupa M, Siitonen O, Laitinen J, Lansimies E. Habitual physical activity, aerobic capacity and metabolic control in patients with newly diagnosed type II diabetes mellitus: effect of a one year diet and exercise intervention. *Diabetologia* 1992; **35**: 340–346.

39. Larsen JJS, Dela F, Kjaer M, Galbo H. The effect of moderate exercise on post prandial glucose homeostasis in NIDDM patients. *Diabetologia* 1997; **40**: 447–453.

40. Lehmann R, Vokac A, Niedermann K, Agosti K, Spinas GA. Loss of abdominal fat and improvement of the cardiovascular risk profile by regular moderate exercise training in patients with NIDDM. *Diabetologia* 1995; **38**: 1313–1319.

41. Boule NG, Haddad E, Kenny GP, Wells GA, Sigal RJ. Effects of exercise on glycaemic control and body mass in type 2 diabetes mellitus. A meta-analysis of controlled clinical trials. *JAMA* 2001; **286**: 1218–1227.

42. Barnard J, Tiffany J, Inkeles SB. Diet and exercise in the treatment of NIDDM. *Diabetes Care* 1994; **17**: 1469–1472.

43. Maiorana A, O'Driscoll G, Goodman C, Taylor R, Green D. Combined aerobic and resistance exercise improves glycaemic control and fitness in type 2 diabetes. *Diabet Res Clin Pract* 2002; **56**: 115–123.

44. Fennicchia LM, Kanaley JA, Azevedo Jr JL, Miller CS, Weinstock RS, Carhart RL, Ploutz-Snyder LL. Influence of resistance exercise training on glucose control in women with type 2 diabetes. *Metabolism* 2004; **53**: 284–289.

45. Holten MK, Zacho M, Gaster M, Carsten J, Wojtaszeski JFP, Dela F. Strength training increase insulin-mediated glucose uptake, GLUT4 content, and insulin signalling in skeletal muscle in patients with type 2 diabetes. *Diabetes* 2004; **53**: 294–305.

46. Eriksson KF, Lindgarde F. Prevention of type 2 (non-insulin dependent) diabetes mellitus by diet and physical exercise: the six year Malmo feasibility study. *Diabetologia* 1991; **34**: 891–898.

47. Schneider SH, Amorosa LF, Khachadurian AK, Ruderman NB. Studies on the mechanism of improved glucose control during regular exercise in type 2 (non-insulin dependent) diabetes mellitus. *Diabetologia* 1984; **26**: 355–360.

48. Krotkiewski M, Loaroth P, Manrwoukas K, Wroblewski Z, Rebuffe-serive M, Holme G, Smith U, Bjorntorp P. Effects of physical training on insulin secretion and effectiveness and glucose metabolism in obesity and type 2 diabetes mellitus. *Diabetologia* 1995; **28**: 881–890.

49. Krotkiewski M, Manrwoukas K, Sjostrom L, SuDivan L, Wetterquist H, Bjorntorp P. Effects of long term physical training on body fat, metabolism and BP in obesity. *Metabolism* 1979; **28**: 650–658.

50. Vu Tran, Weltman A, Glazes G, Mood D. The effects of exercise on plasma lipids and lipoproteins: a meta-analysis of studies. *Med Sci Sport Exercise* 1983; **15**: 393–402.

51. Superko HR. Exercise training, serum lipids, and lipoprotein particle: is there a change threshold. *Med Sci Sport Exercise* 1991; **23**: 677–685.

52. Laws A, Reaven GM. Evidence for an independent relationship between insulin resistance and fasting plasma HDL-cholesterol, triglyceride and insulin concentrations. *J Intern Med* 1992; **232**: 25–30.

53. Van Gaal L, Rillaerts E, Greten W, DeLeeuw I. Relationship of body fat distribution to atherogenic risk in NIDDM. *Diabetes Care* 1988; **11**: 103–106.

54. Ferrannini E, Buzzigoli G, Bonadonna R, Giorico MA, Oleggini M, Graziadei L, Pedrinelli R, Brandi L, Bevilacqua S. Insulin resistance in essential hypertension. *New Engl J Med* 1987; **317**: 350–357.

55. DeFronzo RA. The effect of insulin on renal sodium metabolism. *Diabetologia* 1981; **21**: 165–171.
56. Landsberg L. Diet, obesity and hypertension; an hypothesis involving insulin, the sympathetic nervous system, and adaptive thermogenesis. *Q J Med* 1986; **236**: 1081–1090.
57. Rocchini AP, Katch V, Schork A, Kelch RP. Insulin and blood pressure during weight loss in obese adolescents. *Hypertension* 1987; **10**: 267–273.
58. Schneider SH, Kim HC, Khachandurian AK, Ruderman NB. Impaired fibrinolytic response to exercise in type 2 diabetes: effects of exercise and physical training. *Metabolism* 1988; **37**: 924–929.
59. Gris JC, Schved JF, Aguilar-Martinez P, Amaud A, Sanchez N. Impact of physical training on plasminogen activator inhibitor activity in sedentary men. *Fibrinolysis* 1988; **4** (suppl. 2): 97–98.
60. Juhan Vague I, Alessi MC, Vague P. Increased plasminogen activator inhibitor 1 levels. A possible link between insulin resistance and atherothrombosis. *Diabetologia* 1991; **34**: 457–462.
61. Hamsten A, Wiman B, de Faire U, Blombóck M. Increased plasma levels of a rapid inhibitor of tissue plasminogen activator in young survivors of myocardial infarction. *New Engl J Med* 1985; **313**: 1557–1563.
62. Gray R, Yudkin JS, Patterson D. Plasminogen activator inhibitor: a risk factors for acute myocardial infarction in diabetic patients. *Br Heart J* 1993; **69**: 228–232.
63. Maiorana A, O'Driscoll G, Ceetham C, Dembo L, Stanton K, Goodman C *et al*. The effect of combined aerobic and resistance training on vascular function in type 2 Diabetes. *J Am College Cardiol* 2001; **38**: 860–866.
64. Jenkins AB, Furler SM, Bruce DG, Chisholm DJ. Regulation of hepatic glucose output during moderate exercise in non-insulin dependent diabetes. *Metabolism* 1988; **10**:   966–972.
65. Kjaer M, Hollenbeck CB, Frey-Hewitt B, Galbo H, Haskell W, Reaven GM. Glucoregulation and hormonal responses to maximal exercise in non-insulin dependent diabetes. *J Appl Physiol* 1990; **68**: 2067–2074.
66. Schneider SH, Khachadurian AK, Amoroso LF, Gavras SE, Fineberg SE, Ruderman NB. Abnormal glucoregulation during exercise in type 2 (non-insulin-dependent) diabetes. *Metabolism* 1986; **36**: 1161–1166.
67. Bjorntorp P. Effects of exercise on plasma insulin. *Int J Sports Med* 1981; **2**: 125–129.
68. Bjorntorp P, DeJounge K, Sjostrom L, Sullivan L. The effects of physical training on insulin production in obesity. *Metabolism* 1980; **19**: 631–638.
69. Rosenthal M, Haskell WL, Solomon R, Widstrom A, Reaven GM. Demonstration of a relationship between level of physical training and insulin-stimulated glucose ultilization in normal humans. *Diabetes* 1983; **32**: 408–411.
70. Devlin JT, Hirshman M, Horton ED, Horton ES. Enhanced peripheral and splanchnic insulin sensitivity in NIDDM men after a single bout of exercise. *Diabetes* 1987; **36**:   434–439.
71. Devlin JT, Barlow J, Horton ES. Whole body and regional fuel metabolism during early post-exercise recovery. *Am J Physiol* 1989; **256**: E167–E172.
72. Ivy JL, Holloszy JO. Persistent increase in glucose uptake by rat skeletal muscle following exercise. *Am J Physiol* 1981; **241**: C200–C203.
73. Bogardus C, Ravussin E, Robbins DC, Wolfe DC, Horton ES, Sims EAH. Effects of physical training and diet therapy on carbohydrate metabolism in patients with glucose intolerance and non-insulin dependent diabetes mellitus. *Diabetes* 1984; **33**: 311–318.
74. King AC, Haskell Wl, Taylor CB, Kraemer HC, Debusk RF. Home based exercise training in healthy older men and women. *JAMA* 1991; **266**: 1535–1542.

75. Koivisto VA, Soman V, Conrad P, Hendler R, Nadel E, Felig P. Insulin binding to monocytes in trained athletes: changes in the resting state and after exercise. *J Clin Invest* 1979; **64**: 1011–1015.

76. Dohm GL, Sinha MK, Caro JF. Insulin receptor binding and protein kinase activity in muscles of trained rats. *Am J Physiol* 1987; **252**: E170–E175.

77. Musi N, Fujii N, Hirshman MF, Ekberg I, Froberg S, Ljungqvist O, Thorell A, Goodyear LJ. AMP-activated protein kinase (AMPK) is activated in muscle of subjects with type 2 diabetes during exercise. *Diabetes* 2001; **50**: 921–927.

78. Burnstein R, Polychronakos C, Toews CJ, MacDougall JD, Guyda HJ, Posner BI. Acute reversal of enhanced insulin action in trained athletes. *Diabetes* 1987; **36**: 434–439.

79. Henriksson J. Influence of exercise on insulin sensitivity. *J Cardiovasc Risk* 1995; **2**: 303–309.

80. Koivisto VA, DeFronzo RA. Exercise in the treatment of type 2 diabetes. *Acta Endocrinol* 1984; **262**: 107–111.

81. Borgouts LB, Keizer HA. Exercise and insulin sensitivity: a review. *Int J Sports Med* 1999; **20**: 1–12.

6

The Role of Exercise in the Management of Type 2 Diabetes

Dinesh Nagi

6.1 Introduction

The main goals of treatment in diabetes are the relief of symptoms, prevention and treatment of acute and long-term complications and management of accompanying disorders such as hypertension and dyslipidaemia, reduction of morbidity and mortality and enhancement of quality of life. If physical activity is to be recommended as treatment for type 2 diabetes, it must help to achieve some or ideally most of the therapeutic goals with minimal side effects. Therefore, the risk–benefit ratio of physical activity must be favourable for us to recommend it as a treatment option.

A substantial proportion of patients with newly diagnosed type 2 diabetes have both micro- and macrovascular complications at the time of clinical diagnosis of diabetes.[1,2] This is true whether the disease is diagnosed in those with symptoms[1] or in asymptomatic individuals screened with repeated oral glucose tolerance tests.[2] It is, therefore, of vital importance to also review the impact of physical activity on macro- and microvascular complications of diabetes, while considering its impact on glycaemia and other risk factors. The metabolic syndrome associated with type 2 diabetes includes central obesity, dyslipidaemia and abnormalities of fibrinolysis and coagulation, which contribute to an excess risk of coronary heart disease and hypertension.[3] The relationship of the metabolic syndrome to physical activity is reviewed in more detail in Chapter 3. In Western populations 25–30 per cent of non-diabetic subjects may have features of this syndrome[4] and this proportion is higher in those with type 2 diabetes. Ferrannini et al.[5] found that up

Exercise and Sport in Diabetes, 2nd Edition   Edited by Dinesh Nagi
© 2005 John Wiley & Sons, Ltd.

to two-thirds of the non-diabetic population had one or multiple components of this syndrome with only one-third of individuals being completely free.

Physical inactivity is related to all components of the metabolic syndrome[6,7] and it is therefore logical to see if an increase in physical activity will have beneficial effects. Although it may be important to know that physical activity has benefits in addition to those due to dietary modifications, physical activity is generally recommended in the initial management plan in conjunction with diet.[8] There is evidence that physical activity may improve glucose utilization by mechanisms which differ from those of diet,[9] and the combination of diet and physical activity may be additive or synergistic.[10]

Physical activity is also of benefit in treating dyslipidaemia and hypertension, risk factors which contribute substantially to the excess mortality from macrovascular disease.[11] There is now an established rationale for prescribing physical activity in type 2 diabetes (Table 6.1) and the view that an increase in physical activity may benefit most patients with type 2 diabetes is becoming popular, at least among diabetologists. This is linked to the realization that treatment of hyperglycaemia alone is unlikely to produce benefits in terms of risk reduction in mortality from macrovascular disease.

Table 6.1   Rationale for promoting physical activity in type 2 diabetes

- As an adjunct to diet for initial weight loss
- Aid to help maintain the weight loss
- Loss and redistribution of abdominal fat
- Favourable effect on glycaemic control
- Management of hypertension in diabetes
- Management of dyslipidaemia
- Improvement in general well-being

6.2   Benefits of Regular Physical Activity in Type 2 Diabetes

The benefits of regular physical activity in type 2 diabetes have been known for years and formed the basis of the American Diabetes Association (ADA) recommendations (Table 6.2);[12] they are summarized in Chapter 5.

Table 6.2   ADA recommendations of exercise in type 2 diabetes

- Lowers blood glucose
- Increases insulin sensitivity
- Improves lipid profile
- Promotion of weight loss
- Maintenance of body weight
- Reduction in dose/need for insulin or oral agents

In brief, moderate intensity physical activity, if taken regularly and at frequent intervals, is likely to improve plasma glucose concentration in the short and long term due to beneficial effects on hepatic and peripheral insulin sensitivity. This is not surprising as the exercising muscles use seven to 20 times more glucose than non-exercising muscles.[13] The long-term improvement in glycaemic control is likely to be due to the cumulative effect of repeated bouts of physical activity. It is also suggested that the improvement in fasting plasma glucose may be of larger magnitude in those on diet or oral hypoglycaemic agents than in those treated with insulin.[14] These results indicate that the best time to promote physical activity in subjects with type 2 diabetes is around the time of diagnosis, a time when motivation for behaviour change is generally at its highest in most subjects. There is evidence that increased physical activity in those on drug treatment for diabetes is associated with a reduction, or often discontinuation, of treatment in a substantial proportion of patients.[10,15] Regular physical activity has been shown to be of benefit in promoting weight loss when used in conjunction with diet and may also help to maintain weight loss in the long term.[10,16]

The role of regular physical activity initiated at or around the time of diagnosis of type 2 diabetes in delaying the need for drug treatment needs to be evaluated further. Another potential role of physical activity in the clinical management of type 2 diabetes may be to limit the undesirable weight gain usually associated with initiation of sulfonylurea or insulin treatment, and needs to be investigated.

The benefits of physical activity in type 2 diabetes in relation to its effects on dyslipidaemia and hypertension are of equal importance, as successful modification of these two risk factors has been shown to reduce mortality from macrovascular disease.[17] The results of the United Kingdom Prospective Diabetes Study (UKPDS), published recently, showed that intensive blood glucose control in subjects with type 2 diabetes significantly reduced risk of microvascular complication by 25 per cent. However, the effect on diabetes-related death, and all-cause mortality was small and not significant.[18] Similarly tighter control of blood pressure of less than 144/82 mmHg was also associated with a highly significant reduction in diabetes-related death (32 per cent), strokes (44 per cent) and microvascular disease (37 per cent).[19] The results of UKPDS also showed that, to achieve these benefits, patients have to take a number of tablets for glycaemic control, management of hypertension and lowering cholesterol. Thus it is important to consider the effects of exercise in the context of this important study.

A meta-analysis of the effects of exercise on glycaemic control and body weight concluded that exercise reduces HbA1c by approximately 0.66 per cent, an amount which may be clinically significant in the long run. They did not find any greater weight loss in the exercise group. They found that the differences between exercise and control groups were not mediated by differences in weight, exercise intensity and the volume of exercise.[20] Therefore, exercise does not have to reduce weight to have a beneficial effect on glucose control. If this impact of exercise can be maintained for a sustained period of time, it is likely that the benefits will be significant, considering that an HbA1c reduction of 0.9 per cent seen in the UKPDS reduced complications of diabetes significantly.

Similarly, in a meta-analysis of 25 studies looking at the effects of physical activity on blood pressure, there was an average reduction of 11 and 8 mmHg, respectively, in systolic and diastolic blood pressures. This magnitude of blood pressure reduction may be particularly useful in those with mild hypertension and in early stages of the disease.[21] Again, to put it in the context of UKPDS, a difference of 10 mmHg of systolic and 5 mmHg of diastolic blood pressure, between intensively and less intensively treated groups, was associated with a highly significant impact on the macro- and microvascular complications.

The effects of physical activity on lipids have been discussed in Chapter 4 and involve a reduction in triglyceride and a rise in high-density lipoprotein (HDL) cholesterol, both of which may be related to reduced insulin resistance.[22] There is also some reduction of LDL cholesterol levels as well as an improvement in LDL particle density, thereby making it less atherogenic. The effects of physical activity when combined with diet are more marked than those seen with dietary modification alone. In addition to the specific benefits on risk factors for cardiovascular disease, there are other ancillary benefits (Table 6.3).

Table 6.3 Potential benefits of regular physical activity in type 2 diabetes

- Lowers blood glucose during and after exercise
- Increases insulin sensitivity
- Lowers basal and post prandial insulin levels
- Lowers glycated haemoglobin over long term
- Lowers systolic and diastolic blood pressures
- Quantitative and qualitative changes in circulating lipids
   - lower triglyceride, lower LDL cholesterol, higher HDL cholesterol
   - beneficial effects on LDL density?
- Improves fibrinolysis, lowers plasma fibrinogen
- Other benefits
   - cardiovascular conditioning
   - improves strength
   - improves sense of well-being (physical and psychological)
   - better quality of life

6.3 Effects on Long-Term Mortality

There are no long-term randomized intervention studies assessing the effect of physical activity on total and cardiovascular mortality in subjects with type 2 diabetes. Such studies would have major logistic problems and ethical considerations and therefore they are unlikely to be done. One is, therefore, dependent upon the studies which were non-randomized or on information from meta-analysis of small studies. In the Malmo study, Eriksson et al.,[23] in their 6 year study of an outpatient-based physical activity programme, studied subjects with type 2 diabetes and impaired glucose tolerance. The overall mortality in the whole cohort was 3.3 per cent (230 of 6956 subjects), with an annual mortality figure of 0.5 per cent. The relative risk of death in the treatment cohort with life style interventions (five of 222 subjects) was 0.67, and was not statistically significantly different from the control group. However, no cases of acute myocardial infarction occurred among those who continued with the treatment protocol for a period of 6 years, which is reassuring. The cumulative mortality in subjects with IGT and type 2 diabetes who participated in the program was 3.2 per cent, which was significantly less than those with known diabetes (mortality 11.9 per cent). Clearly, only a limited conclusion can be drawn from this non-randomized study, nevertheless physical activity appears to be safe over a long-term period and may potentially have benefits in terms of lowering mortality. The recent publication of 12 year follow-up from the same study showed in subjects with impaired glucose tolerance (IGT) that lifestyle interventions with diet and exercise achieved mortality rates similar to those of subjects with normal glucose tolerance.[24]

In a meta-analysis of studies investigating the role of physical activity in relation to primary prevention of coronary artery disease in non-diabetic subjects, Berlin and Colditz[25] found that the relative risk of death comparing sedentary vs non-sedentary subjects was 1.9 (95 per cent confidence interval, CI, 1.6–2.2). Their analysis included 27 studies of occupational and eight studies of non-occupational activity.[25] They also suggested that the studies which were methodologically stronger showed a larger benefit. O'Connor et al.[26] analysed 22 randomized studies of rehabilitation following acute myocardial infarct, which included physical activity as part of the rehabilitation programme, and found mortality to be reduced by 20 per cent. The results were also very similar in studies which included physical activity alone as part of rehabilitation. Although these results are from studies performed in non-diabetic subjects, there does not seem to be any good reason why these results should not be applicable to subjects with type 2 diabetes. These observations would suggest that regular physical activity is likely to be of benefit in reducing mortality and prolonging life.

In non-diabetic subjects, regular physical activity is known to improve psychological well-being and overall quality of life.[27] Although there are no studies in subjects with type 2 diabetes in this respect, these benefits are generally perceived by patients to be of equal importance to the effects of physical well being.

6.4 Risks of Physical Activity

Sports injuries

Whether or not subjects with diabetes taking physical activity and engaging in exercise and sport are more prone to musculoskeletal injuries when compared with non-diabetic subjects is unknown. A study with a 3 year follow-up showed that there was an association between sports-related ankle fractures and diabetes and obesity in middle-aged and older individuals.[28] It is unclear if the association of diabetes with ankle fracture during sport is independent of obesity. It is reported that subjects with diabetes are prone to stress fracture of the lower extremities, which may be due to the presence of neuropathy, vascular disease and associated low bone density. Upper extremity injuries may also be more common in subjects with diabetes. This may be due to a higher prevalence of periarthritis of shoulder joints in subjects with diabetes than those without (10.8 vs 2.3 per cent). These problems are frequently bilateral and are unrelated to neuropathy.[29]

Musculoskeletal injuries are related to duration and intensity of physical activity. These may result from chronic, repetitive and high-impact injuries rather than actual trauma. Schneider *et al.*[30] noticed that 12 per cent of subjects participating in formal exercise programmes had some sort of injury, but generally these were minor and did not pose a major problem. However, it is important that these risks are discussed with the patient and appropriate steps taken to avoid them. This can be achieved by setting realistic exercise training goals and by limiting the intensity and duration of any sustained activity, particularly during exercise initiation. An initial period of stretching and warming up and cooling down periods are essential and are highlighted in Chapter 11. Proper footwear and surroundings are also vital to minimize these risks.[12]

Hypoglycaemia

The risk of hypoglycaemia applies to patients with type 2 diabetes who are treated with sulfonylureas or insulin. Hypoglycaemia may occur during or soon after physical activity or it may be delayed for up to 24 h following a single bout of exercise, a fact not generally realized by many patients as well as health professionals.[31] Hypoglycaemia is not an issue in those on diet alone or in those taking metformin or α-glucosidase inhibitors. Physical activity can also potentially cause transient or prolonged hyperglycaemia in type 2 diabetes following extremely strenuous physical activity, but generally in those who are insulin deficient and have poor control of diabetes.[32]

Macrovascular complications

Studies have shown that a large proportion of subjects with type 2 diabetes have complications or physical disability which may be an impediment to physical activity (Table 6.4).[30,33] Samaras *et al.*[33] found that in the non-exercising population up to 15 per cent had diabetic foot disease, stroke or joint disease and 30 per cent had evidence of ischaemic heart disease (IHD). They concluded

Table 6.4 Prevalence of complications (%) in patients with type 2 diabetes volunteering for exercise

Complication	Prevalence (%)
Occult coronary artery disease	11
Intermittent claudication	14
Hypertension	42
Sensory neuropathy	76
Autonomic neuropathy	29
Retinopathy	16
Albuminurea	
before exercise	8
after exercise	29

Adapted from Schneider et al.[30]

that those with IHD may not exercise due to perceived disability or risk or through discouragement by health professionals. Ironically, these subjects are the ones who are likely to benefit most and should be targeted for increasing physical activity.[33] In a feasibility study of exercise in patients aged 60 or over which included 48 subjects with type 2 diabetes, 39 were deemed to be unfit for physical training: 14 were taking antihypertensive medication, seven had symptoms suggestive of angina, seven had asymptomatic changes on ECG and 11 had locomotor dysfunction.[34] The authors concluded that the majority of subjects in that age group could not be recommended for physical training. While 'physical training' may be an unrealistic goal in this group, none of these complications are absolute contraindications to mild or moderate-intensity aerobic physical activity, as long as the general principles of initiating physical activity are followed and individualized advice about the type of physical activity is given.

Worsening of pre-existing cardiovascular disease or unmasking of previously asymptomatic coronary heart disease remains a major concern. Up to 20 per cent of newly diagnosed subjects with type 2 diabetes may already have asymptomatic coronary artery disease.[1,35] Sudden death due to acute myocardial infarction, arrhythmias or intracerebral bleed is much dreaded but exceedingly rare, with a documented incidence of 0–2/1 000 000 h of exercise.[36] This risk is only slightly increased in those with pre-existing heart disease.[37] For detailed discussion on exercise considerations in coronary artery and peripheral vascular disease see the paper by Armen and Smith.[38]

Microvascular complications

In theory, strenuous physical activity may have an adverse effect on microvascular complications associated with diabetes. There is no evidence that moderate-intensity physical activity will have little or no detrimental effect on non-proliferative retinopathy and the risk in patients with proliferative retinopathy is low.[39] However, it is prudent to avoid vigorous physical activity which involves pounding or repeated jarring, weight lifting, high-impact aerobics and activities which involve the Valsalva manoeuvre if there is proliferative retinopathy or vitreous haemorrhage. Exercises such as walking, swimming, low-impact aerobics or stationary cycling seem to be appropriate in these individuals. Those with known retinopathy need to have regular retinal review depending on the severity of retinopathy.[12,39]

Exercise is known to increase albuminuria during and in the period of immediately after exercise, although the long-term implications on diabetic nephropathy are unclear.[40,41] Exercise capacity is often limited in subjects with overt nephropathy *per se* or due to concomitant autonomic neuropathy.[42,43] There seems to be no good reason to restrict low- to moderate-intensity exercise in these subjects, although they should be discouraged from high-intensity strenuous physical activity. It is clearly important that in these subjects appropriate attention is paid to achieving and maintaining good glycaemic and rigorous blood pressure control. Those patients with nephropathy who are already on renal dialysis will have reduced exercise capacity. In addition a majority will have co-existing cardiac involvement. However, exercise benefits should apply equally to these subjects, although careful attention needs to be given to adjusting physical activity programmes to the patient's complications and disabilities to help maintain the patient's functional status.

Patients should be screened for peripheral neuropathy, foot deformity or degenerative joint disease to avoid injury and adequate advice about foot care provided. Those who have significant neuropathy and insensitive feet are more prone to foot ulceration and also fractures, so that weight-bearing exercises such as step exercises and prolonged jogging or walking on a treadmill should be undertaken with care or avoided. Sensory involvement with Charcot arthropathy or foot ulcers is generally considered to be an absolute contraindication for weight-bearing exercises. Non-weight bearing exercises such as cycling, swimming, rowing and arm exercises are more appropriate in these circumstances.

Subjects who have autonomic neuropathy may have a decreased capacity for exercise, especially high-intensity exercise, due to their inadequate cardiovascular response to exercise, such as an increase in heart rate. These subjects may be more prone to episodes of extreme hypo or hypertension following exercise, especially if exercise is vigorous.[42] Postural hypotension may be aggravated and they may be at risk of excess fluid loss through sweating, which may be relevant in hot climates. Recently, it has been suggested that, these subjects may also be prone to silent myocardial ischaemia.[43] Exercise in these individuals needs to be gentle and perhaps is better limited to sessions of short duration. There are no available data on the effects of exercise on long-term progression of autonomic neuropathy.

Despite these potentially detrimental effects of exercise on micro- and macro-vascular complications, the benefits of exercise generally outweigh the risks associated with it.[39] Furthermore, the risks can be minimized or avoided through individualization of physical activity programmes through selection of patients through a proper clinical evaluation. Appropriate advice depending upon age, sex, ethnic and cultural background should be available to all. It seems reasonable to tell those who take no regular physical activity that some physical activity is better than none. Those patients wishing to increase physical activity should be instructed to start with relatively low-intensity exercise and build up gradually as physical conditioning to exercise occurs. Patients should also be instructed to limit the duration of exercise at the outset and report immediately any untoward symptoms. They need to choose physical activity which is enjoyable, causes no financial and physical harm and is easily accessible.

There still is no universal consensus as to the intensity and duration of physical activity which is optimal for health benefits. Emerging evidence over the last decade indicates that physical activity of low to moderate intensity is likely to be beneficial[44] and that a combination of both aerobic and high intensity physical activity may be desirable.[45] The suggested frequency and duration of exercise are given in Table 6.5.

Table 6.5 How much physical activity do we need?

- Three to five times a week, spaced at no more than 48 h interval
- Mild to moderate intensity (aerobic and/or resistance training)
- Duration of 15–60 min per session, with warm-up and cool-down periods of approximately 5 min
- Brisk walking, jogging or running, swimming, bicycling, tennis, badminton, skiing, dancing, etc.

6.5 Conclusions

Physical activity may not be a panacea for all ailments, but has beneficial effects on the physical and psychological well-being of patients and has the potential to improve quality of life. Physical activity has effects on glycaemic control and risk factors for cardiovascular disease which in the long run should translate into improved outcomes with a reduction of mortality and prolongation of life. Evidence suggests that regular physical activity has the potential to benefit most patients with type 2 diabetes and the risk–benefit ratio of physical activity is acceptable. However, there continues to be a large gap between theory and practice and sufficient emphasis is currently not being given to the multiple benefits of physical activity in subjects with type 2 diabetes and to the population in general. The advice about physical activity currently given to patients is minimal, with encouraging words such as 'exercise is good for you', or 'you should try to do more exercise', an approach which is likely to be of little benefit. At present, little effort is being made to assess the exercise habits of these subjects and the feasibility of initiation of regular physical activity in a given individual. With so little formal emphasis on the benefits of physical activity, it is not surprising that there is very little success in modifying this aspect of patient behaviour.

Modification of physical activity remains a complex problem and the challenge which faces us is to find ways to increase the uptake of physical activity. Health professionals need to learn more about attitudes and barriers to exercise in patients and to educate our patients and ourselves about the health benefits of exercise. We should use our existing knowledge to promote physical activity in subjects with type 2 diabetes, most of whom are willing and enthusiastic and need to be given proper education and help in this regard. We urgently need to assess the effectiveness of innovative approaches to increase physical activity.[46] The efforts to promote physical activity in subjects with type 2 diabetes are unlikely to succeed without a substantial input from health professionals involved in diabetes care.

Systems of care to promote physical activity need to be developed and incorporated into our current clinical practice. Such systems of care no doubt will require careful planning, more resources and above all rigorous evaluation to critically review the benefits and cost-effectiveness. The role of diabetes teams in promoting physical activity is discussed in detail in Chapter 12. The success in increasing compliance to exercise and changing behaviour in the long run may be best achieved by structured outpatient-based programmes.

We need structured educational programmes as recommended by National Institute of Clinical Excellence (NICE) in England, to provide initial patient education. These programmes should be designed to prepare individuals to exercise safely on their own by choosing activities which fit into their daily lifestyle. Education thus provided should help allay fears and anxieties about exercise, so that they can continue exercising on their own. However, regular and frequent contact with health professionals may be desirable in some individuals to maintain optimum physical activity levels.

References

1. UK Prospective Diabetes Study 6. Complications in newly diagnosed type 2 patients and their associations with different clinical and biochemical risk factors. UKPDS Group. *Diabet Res* 1990; **13**: 1–11.
2. Nagi DK, Pettitt DJ, Bennett PH, Klein R, Knowler WC. Diabetic retinopathy assessed by fundus photography in Pima Indians with impaired glucose tolerance and NIDDM. *Diab Med* 1997; **14**: 449–456.
3. Reaven GM. Role of insulin resistance in human disease. *Diabetes* 1988; **37**: 1595–1607.
4. DeFronzo RA, Ferrannini E. Insulin resistance: a multifaceted syndrome responsible for NIDDM, obesity, hypertension, dyslipidaemia and atherosclerotic vascular disease. *Diabetes Care* 1991; **14**: 173–194.

5. Ferrannini E, Haffner, Mitchell BD, Stern MP. Hyperinsulinaemia: the key feature of a cardiovascular and metabolic syndrome. *Diabetologia* 1991; **34**: 416–422.

6. Paffenbarger RS, Wing AL, Hyde RT, Jung DL. Physical activity and the incidence of hypertension in college alumni. *Am J Epidemiol* 1983; **117**: 245–257.

7. Siscovick DS, Laporte RE, Newman JM. The disease specific benefits and risks of physical activity and exercise. *Public Hlth Rep* 1985; **100**: 180–188.

8. National Institutes of Health. Consensus development conference on diet and exercise in non-insulin-dependent diabetes mellitus. *Diabetes Care* 1987; **10**: 639–644.

9. Bogardus C, Ravussin E, Robbins DC, Wolfe DC, Horton ES, Sims EAH. Effects of physical training and diet therapy on carbohydrate metabolism in patients with glucose intolerance and non-insulin dependent diabetes mellitus. *Diabetes* 1984; **33**: 311–318.

10. Wing RR, Epstein LH, Paternostro-Bayles M, Kriska A, Nowalk MP, Gooding W. Exercise in a behavioral weight control programme for obese patients with type II diabetes. *Diabetologia* 1988; **31**: 902–909.

11. Panzram G. Mortality and survival in type 2 (non-insulin-dependent) diabetes mellitus. *Diabetologia* 1987; **30**: 123–131.

12. American Diabetes Association. Clinical practice recommendations. Diabetes mellitus and exercise. *Diabetes Care* 1998; **21** (suppl. 1): S41–S44.

13. Wahren J, Felig P, Ahlborg G, Jorfeldt L. Glucose metabolism during leg exercise in man. *J Clin Invest* 1971; **50**: 2715–2725.

14. Barnard J, Tiffany J, Inkeles SB. Diet and exercise in the treatment of NIDDM. *Diabetes Care* 1994; **17**: 1469–1472.

15. Heath GW, Leonard BE, Wilson RH, Kendrick JS, Powell KE. Community-based exercise intervention: Zuni diabetes project. *Diabetes Care* 1987; **10**: 579–583.

16. Lehmann R, Vokac A, Niedermann K, Agosti K, Spinas GA. Loss of abdominal fat and improvement of the cardiovascular risk profile by regular moderate exercise training in patients with NIDDM. *Diabetologia* 1995; **38**: 1313–1319.

17. Collins R, Petro R, MacMahon S. Blood pressure stroke, and coronary heart disease. II. Effects of short-term reductions in blood pressure: an overview of the unconfounded randomized drug trials in an epidemiological context. *Lancet* 1990; **335**: 827–838.

18. UK Prospective Diabetes Study (UKPDS) Group. Intensive blood-glucose control with sulphonylurea or insulin compared with conventional treatment and risk of complications in patients with type 2 diabetes (UKPDS 33). *Lancet* 1998; **352**: 837–853.

19. UK Prospective Diabetes Study (UKPDS) Group. Tight blood pressure control and risk of macrovascular complications in type 2 diabetes (UKPDS 38). *Br Med J* 1998; **317**: 703–713.

20. Boule NG, Haddad E, Kenny GP, Wells GA, Sigal RJ. Effects of exercise on glycaemic control and body mass in type 2 diabetes mellitus. A meta-analysis of controlled clinical trials. *JAMA* 2001; **286**: 1218–1227.

21. Hagberg JM. Exercise, fitness and hypertension. In Bouchard C (ed.), *Exercise, Fitness and Health: a Consensus of Current Knowledge*. Champaign, IL: Human Kinetics, 1990.

22. Eriksson J, Taimela S, Koivisto VA. Exercise and the metabolic syndrome. *Diabetologia* 1997; **40**: 125–135.

23. Eriksson KF, Lindgarde F. Prevention of type 2 (non-insulin dependent) diabetes mellitus by diet and physical exercise: the six year Malmo feasibility study. *Diabetologia* 1991; **34**: 891–898.

24. Eriksson KF, Lindgarde F. No excess 12-year mortality in men with impaired glucose tolerance who participated in Malmo preventive trail with diet and exercise. *Diabetologia* 1998; **41**: 1010–1017.

25. Berlin JA, Colditz GA. A meta analysis of physical activity in the prevention of coronary heart disease. *Am J Epidemiol* 1990; **132**: 612–628.
26. O'Connor GT, Buring JE, Yusaf S, Guldhaber SZ, Olmstead EM, Barger RS, Hennekens CH. An overview of randomized trials of rehabilitation with exercise after myocardial infarction. *Circulation* 1989; **80**: 234–244.
27. McAuley E. Physical activity and psychological outcomes. In: Bouchard C, Shepard RG, Stephens T (eds), *Physical Activity, Fitness and Health: International Proceedings and Consensus Statement*. Champaign, IL: Human Kinetics, 1992; 551–568.
28. Daly PJ, Fitzgerald RH Jr, Melton LJ, Ilstrup DM. Epidemiology of ankle fractures in Rochester, Minnesota. *Acta Orthop Scand* 1987; **58**: 539–544.
29. Bridgeman JF. Periarthritis of shoulder and diabetes mellitus. *Am Rheum Dis* 1972; **31**: 69–72.
30. Schneider SH, Khachadurian AK, Amorosa LF, Clemow L, Ruderman NB. Ten-year experience with an exercise-based outpatient life-style modification program in the treatment of diabetes mellitus. *Diabetes Care* 1992; **15** (suppl. 4): 1800–1810.
31. MacDonald MJ. Post-exercise late-onset hypoglycaemia in insulin-dependent diabetic patients. *Diabetes Care* 1987; **10**: 584–588.
32. Mitchell TH, Gebrehiwot A, Abraham G, Schiffrin A, Leiter A, Marless EB. Hyperglycaemia after intense exercise in IDDM subjects during continuous subcutaneous insulin infusion. *Diabetes Care* 1988; **11**: 311–317.
33. Samaras K, Ashwell S, Mackintosh A-M, Campbell LV, Chisholm DJ. Exercise in NIDDM: are we missing the point? *Diab Med* 1996; **13**: 780–781.
34. Skarfors ET, Wegener TA, Lithell H, Selinus I. Physical training as a treatment for type II (non-insulin dependent) diabetes in elderly men. *Diabetologia* 1987; **30**: 930–933.
35. Chiariello M. Silent myocardial ischaemia in patients with diabetes mellitus. *Circulation* 1996; **93**: 2089–2091.
36. Haskell WL. Cardiovascular complications during exercise training of cardiac patients. *Circulation* 1978; **57**: 920–924.
37. Debusk RF, Valdez R, Houston, N, Haskell W. Cardiovascular responses to dynamic and static efforts soon after myocardial infarction. *Circulation* 1978; **58**: 368–375.
38. Armen J, DO, Smith BW. Exercise considerations in coronary artery disease, peripheral vascular disease and diabetes mellitus. *Clin Sports Med* 2003; **22**: 123–133.
39. Devlin J, Ruderman N. Diabetes and exercise: the risk–benefit profile revissisted. In Devlin J, Shneider SH (eds), *Handbook of Exercise in Diabetes*. Alexandria, VA: American Diabetes Association, 2002; 17–20.
40. Mogensen CE, Vittinghus E. Urinary albumin excretion during exercise in juvenile diabetes. *Scand J Clin Lab Invest* 1975; **35**: 295–300.
41. Viberti GC, Jarrett RJ, McCartney M, Keen H. Increased glomerular permeability to albumin induced by exercise in diabetic subjects. *Diabetologia* 1978; **14**: 293–300.
42. Hilsted J, Galbo H, Christensen NJ. Impaired cardiovascular responses to graded exercise in diabetic autonomic neuropathy. *Diabetes* 1979; **28**: 313–319.
43. Vinik A, Erbo T. Neuropathy. In Devlin J, Schneider SH (eds), *Handbook of Exercise in Diabetes*. Alexandria, VA: American Diabetes Association, 2002; 463–496.
44. Blair SN, Kohl HW, Gordon NF, Paffenbarger RS. How much physical activity is good for health. *A Rev Public Hlth* 1992; **13**: 99–126.
45. ACMS/ADA. Joint position statement: diabetes mellitus and exercise. *Med Sci Sports Exercise* 1997; **29**(12): i–iv.
46. Marcus BH, Simkin LR. The transtheoretical model: application to exercise behaviour. *Med Sci Sports Exercise* 1994; **26**: 1400–1404.

7
Exercise in Children and Adolescents

Diarmuid Smith, Alan Connacher, Ray Newton and Chris Thompson

7.1 Introduction

Physical activity is an intrinsic part of everyday life for children and young adults and sporting prowess contributes greatly to the prestige accorded by young people to their peers. Young people consistently place sportsmen and women highly in the pantheon of those they respect and wish to emulate, a relationship which is well recognized by advertising agencies, who use sportsmen and women to endorse a huge range of products from designer clothes and deodorants to junk food and beverages. In contrast, lack of sporting ability or failure of young people to participate in sporting activities can lead to social isolation and loss of self-confidence. Exercise in children and young adults with insulin-dependent (type 1) diabetes mellitus can lead to profound metabolic disturbances, occasionally leading to hyperglycaemia and ketosis or, more frequently, to hypoglycaemia, which can detract from the enjoyment of exercise and reduce confidence to participate, a sequence of events which compounds the sense of loneliness which is experienced by many young people with diabetes. The tragedy of such a scenario is that it need not be so; with a little care, education and organization, people with type 1 diabetes can participate fully in almost any form of exercise. Moreover, as evidence accumulates that regular exercise in early life can confer protection against vascular events in later life, young patients should be actively encouraged to include physical activity in their normal daily routine, in very much the way that they are currently given dietary advice or education about blood glucose monitoring or insulin adjustment.

Exercise and Sport in Diabetes, 2nd Edition   Edited by Dinesh Nagi
© 2005 John Wiley & Sons, Ltd.

In this chapter we describe the pitfalls for young people with type 1 diabetes when they exercise and the strategies adopted to avoid those pitfalls. We also discuss the difficulties in encouraging young people to take regular exercise and the structures, such as camps and courses, within which the adaptations necessary for safe participation in sporting activities are provided. The greater part of our experience with sporting activities has been derived from our association with the annual camp run at Firbush Point Field Centre on the shores of Loch Tay, Scotland. Much of the practical advice included in the chapter has been developed from involvement with young people with diabetes who attend this camp. We therefore describe the structure and philosophy of this camp in order to put into context the attitudes to sport and diabetes which we espouse.

7.2   Metabolic Effects of Exercise

The physiology of exercise is covered in some detail in Chapter 1. Exercise causes a dramatic increase in muscle glucose utilization, and the need for a steady supply of substrate for energy generation. The main substrate is glucose in exercise of short duration, and this is derived from increased hepatic glycogenolysis. During sustained exercise, gluconeogenesis from lactate, alanine and glycerol assumes greater importance.[1] In the non-diabetic human, secretion of insulin from the pancreas is suppressed during exercise and there is a rise in plasma catecholamines,[2] growth hormone and glucocorticoids.[3] This creates a hormonal milieu which allows mobilization of free fatty acids from triglycerides, breakdown of hepatic glycogen stores, stimulation of gluconeogenesis and maintenance of constant plasma glucose concentrations. Blood glucose concentrations remain steady throughout prolonged exercise and for some hours after cessation of exercise.

In people with type 1 diabetes who are exercising, the presence of their usual circulating levels of insulin inhibits hepatic glycogenolysis and gluconeogenesis, which may cause blood glucose levels to fall rapidly into the hypoglycaemic range. A reduction in insulin dosage, or extra carbohydrate consumption, or both, is required shortly before starting to exercise. On the other hand, if insulin levels are reduced too much or stopped altogether, and blood sugars are elevated, exercise can produce a dramatic increase in hyperglycaemia. This may progress to ketosis, rising blood lactate and pyruvate levels,[4] and osmotic symptoms of hyperglycaemia, fatigue, muscle cramps and poor athletic performance. The potential for development of ketosis during exercise in the situation of insulin deficiency is of sufficient importance that the American Diabetes Association position statement on exercise and type 1 diabetes (Table 7.1) specifically advises against exercise in the setting of hyperglycaemia and ketosis.[5]

There is evidence that exercise programmes can substantially increase insulin sensitivity in young people with diabetes with a fall in daily insulin requirements,

Table 7.1 American Diabetes Association guidelines for exercise in diabetes, as derived from the position statement (1990)

1. Use proper footwear, and, if appropriate, other protective equipment
2. Avoid exercise in extreme heat or cold
3. Inspect feet daily and after exercise
4. Avoid exercise during periods of poor metabolic control

but no overall improvement in glycaemic control, as measured by glycated haemoglobin.[6] This lack of improvement in glycaemic control may be partly related to increased carbohydrate intake in order to avoid hypoglycaemia, as many young people eat considerably more around the time of exercise.

It may also relate to the potential for exercise to cause metabolic instability, leading to both hyperglycaemia and hypoglycaemia. There is a need for careful adjustment of insulin dosage and carbohydrate intake, which can, given the erratic nature of teenage life and the random occurrence of the opportunity to partake in exercise, cause management difficulties for many young adults.

7.3 Attitudes to Exercise in Young Adults with Type 1 Diabetes

The role of the school is very important in encouraging participation in sport and exercise, and the attitude of the school to the child with diabetes can have a crucial effect on the child's motivation to become involved in sport. Many children play sports at home with friends but it is in school sports lessons that they are first exposed to a wide spectrum of sporting activities, and the school team is usually the first taste of competitive sport. Although it is now rare, there are still teenagers who report that they were discouraged or even banned from taking part in games lessons in school because of their diabetes. This results in a decrease in confidence and self-worth which can take years to correct. The British Diabetic Association has played a major role in improving knowledge of, and attitudes towards, diabetes in schools over recent years. Teacher training courses now cover basic medical knowledge of diabetes and fear of the condition is gradually subsiding in schools. Sporting clubs tend to be very variable in their attitudes to people with diabetes, but many of the traditional prejudices are breaking down, in part because of publicity and pressure from national diabetes associations, but largely because successful participation in sport by people with diabetes is more widely recognized.

As a child progresses towards the teenage years, exercise traditionally assumes a more central and ritualized role in daily life, although there is evidence, as we embrace the computer lifestyle, that physical exercise is declining in the teenage years. In a survey of 50 children and teenagers with type 1 diabetes, most took part in similar levels of physical exertion to non-diabetic controls, although fewer diabetic children were involved in team sports, suggesting a difficulty in mixing with other children for the purposes of exercise.[7] There is a tendency for decreased participation in sport as children get older.[8] The temptation for teenagers with diabetes to lose contact with regular exercise because of the burden of extra preparation and precautions which they must take is all the greater. Some young people with diabetes are sufficiently well organized and motivated to incorporate exercise into their daily routine, but most need extra motivation.

In the setting of an outpatient clinic, this type of motivation is difficult to achieve. The independent practice of all the authors is to include exercise, along with diet and insulin, as part of the triad of principles which contribute to good glycaemic control and a healthy lifestyle. This entails taking a positive attitude to asking about exercise, discussing the alterations of diet and insulin which are necessary to accommodate successful participation, and encouraging continued involvement. At the time of diagnosis of diabetes, we foster the attitude that patients can continue to participate in exercise and live a normal life – often before diet and insulin injections are even mentioned. The emphasis is very much on minimizing the negative aspects of the effects of diabetes on exercise by giving comprehensive advice about avoidance of hypoglycaemia, while maximizing the benefits of fitness and socializing. The positive aspects of exercise can be demonstrated very clearly in the setting of the out-of-clinic activities. The examples of famous sportsmen such as Danny McGrain (Glasgow Celtic and Scotland), Gary Mabbut (Tottenham Hotspur and England) and Steve Redgrave (Olympic Gold Medal winner), who have achieved high levels of success in prominent sports despite the perceived disadvantage of insulin-dependent diabetes, are often helpful in demonstrating that people with diabetes can and do join in sporting activities and exercise.

Many youngsters who are insufficiently persuaded of the benefits – or safety – of exercise when advised within the slightly forbidding and hierarchical atmosphere of a hospital clinic feel much more relaxed in circumstances where their peers also have diabetes and understand what a 'hypo' is and how to treat it. Out-of-clinic events are thus perceived as a very safe context within which to start or resume exercise by young people with diabetes. The presence of medical staff helps to engender the confidence to try activities which are new or demanding, but it is the knowledge that their experience of having diabetes is shared with others which is probably a more powerful factor in the creation of a secure environment. In this respect, the availability of diabetic camps is an invaluable adjunct to traditional, hospital-based diabetes care, and in particular the fostering of the attitude that regular exercise is important to glycaemic control, physical fitness and general well-being. The first diabetes camp was opened in Michigan, USA in 1925, whereas Diabetes UK has been funding and administering camps for young adults with diabetes since 1936 and well over 100 000 children and young adults have now attended these camps. In Ireland, diabetes camps have been running for young adults since 1997, and have expanded to incorporate highly challenging expeditions to Kilimanjaro, the Canadian Rockies and Machu Pichu.

While the main aim of diabetic camps is simply to provide a happy and enjoyable holiday, the development of social skills[9] and the ability to attain independent control of diabetes are also regarded as important. As nearly all camps contain some element of sport or exercise, the knowledge and practical experience of adjusting diet and insulin to cope with exercise are skills naturally developed as camps progress. The experience of young people attending camps is almost invariably positive,[10] with enthusiasm for the positive attitudes encouraged at camps being shared by the parents.[11] Some specialized camps have included formal fitness programmes[12] or have had well-defined physical objectives,[13] but most simply provide the opportunity and environment conducive to the safe enjoyment of a wide variety of sports and outdoor activities.

7.4 The Firbush Camp

The Firbush Point Field Centre on Loch Tay, Scotland, is run by the Department of Physical Education, University of Edinburgh. Since 1983 it has played host to an annual one-week diabetes outdoor activity holiday for young adults between the ages of 16 and 22 years. The Firbush Programme embraces the traditional aim of diabetes camps, to provide a secure environment in which young people with diabetes can enjoy activities, socialize with other people with diabetes and take the educational opportunity to learn about diabetes and its management. It also seeks to harness the benefits of association between young adults in order to allow those who are confident and independent to give help and encouragement to those less able to cope with diabetic life.[14] Young people with diabetes attend from throughout Britain and Ireland; some respond to advertisements in the Diabetes UK journal, *Balance*, and some are referred on from their clinic doctors or specialist nurses. The activities offered include hillwalking, kayaking, windsurfing, sailing, mountain biking and abseiling. Fully qualified instructors teach the techniques necessary for the activities and a medical team comprising both doctors and specialist nurses is available for advice and troubleshooting, and for organizing educational exercises such as small group discussions and large group seminars.

The initial aims of the Firbush Youth Diabetes Project were to train a cadre of committed young people with diabetes who would then be in a position to set up local diabetes groups to provide a support network for teenagers with diabetes throughout Britain. In the early years of the camp this ethos proved to be exceptionally important in disseminating self-confidence in young people with diabetes, although this role has assumed less importance with the expansion of interest in the formation of local youth diabetes groups. The Firbush Camp has adopted more the role of a medium within which young people with diabetes can learn more about diabetes through discussion of diabetes issues with other youngsters and the adjustment of insulin and diet to meet the demands of an intensely physical week.

Many of the young people attending Firbush have never previously attempted the sports and activities which are available at the centre. The presence of a trained medical team providing back-up to high-quality activity instructors gives them the confidence to attempt many sports which they would never have otherwise contemplated. The atmosphere and team spirit generated in an 'all-diabetes' environment strengthens the sense of security and increases the motivation to participate. Over the last few years, the medical records from Firbush justify this confidence, as very few mishaps have been recorded. The opportunity to engage in physical activity with other people with diabetes is an important aspect of the success and popularity of Firbush, as well as similar camps such as the one run by Rowan Hillson in Eskdale.[13] In this environment there is no longer a stigma associated with insulin injections, blood testing and hypos, and there is an ability to discuss coping strategies with other youngsters with diabetes – medical staff are often regarded as knowledgeable but impractical. Young people develop the confidence to experiment with insulin and diet in order to accommodate exercise into their daily routine.

The ability to learn from other people with diabetes is enormous and most camps will utilize the non-hierarchical, unthreatening atmosphere of a camp to include educational group meetings. The Firbush camp uses a combination of daily small discussion groups and large group forums, whereas the Irish camps concentrate solely on small discussion groups. The Firbush camps invariably have facilitators with medical or nursing backgrounds, but the Irish camps also offer trained facilitators with diabetes such that campers can elect to attend discussion groups with no medical staff present. The groups allow informal discussion of a range of subjects. A group from Turkey reported that nutritional and diabetic knowledge improved after attendance at two camps,[15] although with no improvement in glycaemic control. The Italian experience has been similar, with reported improvement and knowledge, but improvement in HbA1c only in those who attended monthly follow-up meetings with their parents.[16] The American Diabetes Association position statement[17] emphasizes the educational potential of camps and suggests a range of educational topics, including insulin injection techniques and dose adjustment, blood glucose monitoring, recognition of hypos and ketosis, sexual activity and preconception issues, complications, the importance of control, new therapies, carbohydrate counting and problem-solving skills.

The camp should be led by an individual with expertise in managing diabetes and in handling diabetic emergencies such as hypoglycaemia and ketosis. Preferably, the camp leader should also have experience in participating in previous camps. The camp leader is ultimately responsible for the medical care of children attending camps. A mixture of expertise is valuable in the team. Nursing staff are essential components of the team and young campers often consider nurses more approachable than doctors. The value to junior doctors of attending a camp has been stressed[17] and can be an extremely valuable educational process in their training.[18] Attendance at a diabetic camp is now an integral recommendation of specialist training in Ireland. Dieticians have also an important role in planning camp menus, although it is not necessary for their inclusion in the team. In Ireland, dieticians attend the camps as integral members of the team.

It is important that the medical team is familiar with the treatment of diabetes emergencies before the camp begins. It is also preferable for the team to meet before the camp starts to discuss the programme, the house rules, camp policies towards alcohol and non-participation and to familiarize themselves with the medical kit and procedures for dealing with emergencies. The pre-camp meeting is also useful to go through the biographies of the attending campers and highlight any likely problems. The American Diabetes Association has issued a useful Camp Implementation Guide,[19] which documents some of the camp policies which are recommended by that association. Our adaptation of their suggested medical management plan includes:

- general diabetes management;

- insulin injections/pump therapy and blood glucose monitoring;

- timing and content of meals and snacks;

- routine and special activities;

- hypoglycaemia and treatment;

- hyperglycaemia/ketosis and treatment;

- assessment and treatment of intercurrent illness;

- pharmacy contents, site and availability;

- arrangements with local medical services;

- psychological issues and policies towards individuals who find it difficult to integrate or make friends;

- incident/accident reporting;

- when to notify parents or guardians;

- policies towards camp closure and returning home.

7.5   Precautions During Exercise

Hypoglycaemia may occur during physical activity, but in addition it has recently been noted that exercise quite commonly increases insulin sensitivity for a matter of hours after activity has ceased, leading to the development of late hypoglycaemia.

Hypoglycaemia during exercise

The fall in blood glucose concentration which accompanies exercise frequently produces hypoglycaemic symptoms, which are usually mild and easily dealt with, but which are occasionally severe, particularly if they are initially overlooked. The adrenergic surge during exercise produces symptoms which may be difficult to distinguish from hypoglycaemia – or ignored in the excitement of the moment. Frost et al.[20] found an incidence of 85 clinical episodes of hypoglycaemia in 38 children in the first 2 weeks of consecutive diabetic camps. Although most episodes are mild and readily treated, severe hypoglycaemia is not uncommon, and fits have been reported.[21] The likelihood of hypoglycaemia during exercise is influenced by a variety of parameters, including the following.

Pre-exercise blood glucose concentration

Hypoglycaemia is very likely if the blood glucose concentration is $<7\,\mathrm{mmol\,l^{-1}}$ before exercise, and advice should be given to take extra rapidly absorbed carbohydrate if this is the case.

Pre-exercise plasma insulin concentration

Although plasma insulin concentrations are not measured before exercise, the greater the subcutaneous bolus injected before exercise the greater the likelihood of hypoglycaemia during, or after, the period of exercise. Frost et al.,[20] in the setting of a diabetic camp, found that hypoglycaemia occurs far more frequently when the total daily insulin dose exceeds $0.7\,\mathrm{units\,kg^{-1}}$ body weight. At the Firbush camp, we give broad advice to reduce daily insulin dosage by 25 per cent from day 1 of camp activities, although there is a wide variation in individual insulin requirements throughout the week of activities. In practice, the mean reduction in insulin is 25–30 per cent of pre-camp dosage, and mild hypoglycaemia is still common (Table 7.2).

Our experiences at Firbush are very similar to those of the Auckland group, who run a summer camp in New Zealand for a slightly younger age group (7–12 years).

Table 7.2 Daily insulin doses and frequency of mild hypoglycaemia at Firbush camp 1992–1995

Day	1	2	3	4	5	6	7
Insulin dose (percentage of usual daily dose)	83.7	74.1	70.7	73.1	72.4	70.1	69.2
Total hypos (grades 1 and 2 only)	201	66	81	92	89	87	56

This group found that hypoglycaemia was common, particularly during the first few days of camp, despite a mean reduction in daily insulin dose of 33 per cent.[22] There was a deliberate policy not to increase carbohydrate intake in this camp. This is in direct contrast to our own policy to allow free access to carbohydrate, and to encourage an increase in carbohydrate intake to counteract the increase in energy expenditure which particularly occurs during prolonged exercise. This approach is used by other groups, and during a winter skiing camp a Finnish group reported a mean increase in calorie intake of 31 per cent, although the daily insulin dose was reduced only by a mean of 11.8 per cent.[12]

Nature of exercise; duration and intensity

The frequency and severity of hypoglycaemia increases with the duration and intensity of exercise. Short bursts of intense activity, such as squash or aerobics, are particularly likely to cause hypoglycaemia, but in practice patients successfully anticipate the likelihood of hypoglycaemia in such sports, and prevent hypos by increasing carbohydrate intake and reducing insulin before they exercise. It is often sustained exercise which catches patients unawares: at Firbush, the activities most commonly associated with frequent and severe hypos are hillwalking, canoeing and mountain biking, which are all sports typified by intense exercise of long duration.

Extremes of temperature

Hot weather causes vasodilatation and the increased skin blood flow causes more rapid absorption of insulin from subcutaneous depots, with a consequently greater risk of hypoglycaemia. The effect of cold is even more dramatic; low temperatures are associated with shivering, which, in order to induce thermogenesis, increases metabolic rate and fuel consumption, with a resultant risk of hypoglycaemia.[23] Cold-induced hypoglycaemia is a particular feature of water sports such as canoeing and windsurfing, and extra vigilance is needed when supervising these sports, especially in adverse weather conditions. The implications of severe hypoglycaemia when a camper is on a windsurfer or in a canoe in white water conditions are significant and we do not recommend participation in these sports without full awareness of the prevention of hypoglycaemia, good availability of carbohydrate and close supervision by qualified personnel.

Delayed hypoglycaemia

The phenomenon of hypoglycaemia with onset some hours after the cessation of exercise has been recognized for some time, but only a minority of young adults with type 1 diabetes receive formal advice about the risks of delayed hypoglycaemia, or the strategies to avoid it. In one prospective study of 300 children and teenagers attending a paediatric diabetic clinic, 15 per cent had late post-exercise hypoglycaemia in a 2-year follow-up period, with more than half of the cases resulting in loss of consciousness or seizures, and requiring treatment with intravenous glucose or subcutaneous glucagon.[24] In a 4-year period at the Firbush camp, 1992–1995, we witnessed six episodes of severe (grade 4) hypoglycaemia, all of which occurred in the evening, several hours after exercise had ceased. In all cases, the preceding activity had consisted of sustained exercise – hillwalking or canoeing – with several minor (grade 1 or 2) hypos during the day. The daytime hypoglycaemic reactions may be significant in this respect, as there is now evidence to suggest that frequent hypoglycaemia can reduce awareness that blood glucose concentration is falling (see below).

Nocturnal hypos after exercise are extremely disconcerting to young people with diabetes. Mild hypoglycaemia occurring during exercise is perceived as predictable, easily detected and straightforward to deal with, often without significant interference with participation. Delayed hypoglycaemia is seen as less predictable and, because it typically occurs during the night, more frightening and difficult to deal with. We regard specific advice about the existence of delayed-onset hypoglycaemia, and its prevention, as essential components of our instruction package for young people with diabetes who wish to partake in regular exercise. In particular, we stress the importance of a good snack and monitoring of blood glucose concentration before going to bed; a blood glucose concentration of $<7 \, \text{mmol} \, \text{l}^{-1}$ is highly predictive of nocturnal hypoglycaemia and should prompt extra carbohydrate intake.

The mechanisms behind the development of delayed hypoglycaemia are complex. During even brief exercise, hepatic glucose output increases by up to 5-fold in order to supply sufficient glucose to keep pace with increased utilization by muscle.[25] This can lower liver glycogen to such an extent that it can take up to 2 days to replete glycogen stores.[1] Exercise also lowers muscle glycogen stores, which must be replaced at the expense of blood glucose. Exercise increases insulin sensitivity, and this effect can be sustained for up to 12 h or more after exertion.[6]

To counteract these effects it is often necessary to reduce the dose of long-acting insulin after sustained exercise as well as increasing carbohydrate intake. Alcohol intake significantly increases the likelihood of delayed hypoglycaemia, such that older teenagers and young adults should be specifically warned about the effect of alcohol intake. This is particularly important in the context of social pressures to travel straight from pitch to pub.

In addition to the tendency of physical activity to cause both early and late hypoglycaemia, there is the problem of reduced hypoglycaemia awareness. It has recently been shown that even mild hypoglycaemia is capable of completely abolishing the sympathetic warning signs associated with severe hypoglycaemia occurring in the subsequent 24 h.[26] The need for careful precautions to guard against delayed hypoglycaemia cannot be over-emphasized.

Foot care

It is important to stress the value of foot care in people with type 1 diabetes who exercise regularly. The American Diabetes Position statement[5] (Table 7.1) emphasizes the crucial importance of proper foot care to participation in sport and exercise. Good quality footwear – whether running shoes, football boots or walking boots – which is comfortable and appropriate to the exercise in question is essential for the safe enjoyment of sports. Similarly, high-quality hosiery which can cushion the feet against repetitive trauma is recommended (e.g. Thorlo[1] socks). Regular foot examination should be incorporated into the routine of preparation for exercise and care after completion of exercise. Prolonged exercise may cause blistering of the feet, and supplies of blister packs should be carried, particularly on hillwalking expeditions.

Insulin injections

The influence of the site of insulin injection on exercise-induced hypoglycaemia has been the topic of some debate. It has been reported that leg exercise, in the form of cycling, can increase the rate of insulin absorption,[27] and that hypoglycaemia might be avoided by injecting into non-exercising sites such as the abdomen,[28] although other workers have disputed these findings.[29] We have not been able to show any practical problems with any injection site in the Firbush Camp. Older data from Firbush indicated that only a small minority of young people with diabetes actually injected soluble insulin 30 min before meals, although as more teenagers move towards the use of insulin analogues, the implications of this behaviour pattern is less important.

7.6　Summary

Exercise is an integral part of teenage life. In addition to the benefits of physical fitness and reduced cardiovascular risk which exercise confers on all participants, in diabetes regular exercise lowers cholesterol, increases insulin sensitivity and leads to a reduction in insulin requirements. Most importantly, exercise provides an important medium for the young person with diabetes to integrate fully into normal life in young adulthood. Although precautions are required to participate safely in sports, good education and motivation from the medical team can help the young person with diabetes to participate in almost any sporting activity and achieve standards equal to those achieved by people without diabetes.

References

1. Wahren J, Felig P, Hagenfeldt L. Physical exercise and fuel homeostasis in diabetes mellitus. *Diabetologia* 1978; **14**: 213–222.
2. Christensen NJ, Galbo H, Hansen JF, Hesse B, Richter EA. Catecholamines and exercise. *Diabetes* 1979; **28** (suppl. 1): 58–62.
3. Hartley LH, Mason JW, Hogan RP. Multiple hormonal responses to prolonged exercise in relation to physical training. *J Appl Physiol* 1972; **33**: 602–606.
4. Berger M *et al.* Metabolic and hormonal effects of muscular exercise in juvenile type diabetes. *Diabetologia* 1977; **18**: 355–365.
5. American Diabetes Association. Diabetes and exercise; position statement. *Diabetes Care* 1990; **13**: 804–805.
6. Landt KW, Campaigne BA, James FW, Sperling MA. Effects of exercise training on insulin sensitivity in adolescents with type I diabetes. *Diabetes Care* 1985; **8**: 461–465.
7. Greene SA, Thompson CJ. Exercise. In *Childhood and Adolescent Diabetes*, Kelnar CJH (ed.). London: Chapman & Hall, 1995; 283–293.
8. Boreham C, Savage JM, Primrose D, Cran G, Strain J. Coronary risk factors in school children. *Arch Dis Child* 1993; **68**: 182–186.
9. Thompson CJ, Greene SA, Newton RW. Camps for diabetic children and teenagers. In *Childhood and Adolescent Diabetes*, Kelner CJH (ed.). London: Chapman & Hall, 1995; 483–492.
10. McGraw RK, Travis LG. Psychological effects of a special summer camp on juvenile diabetics. *Diabetes* 1973; **22**: 217–224.
11. Vyas S, Mullee MA, Kinmonth A-L. British Diabetic Association holidays – what are they worth? *Diab Med* 1987; **5**: 89–92.
12. Akerblom HK, Koivukangas T, Ilkka J. Experience from a winter camp for teenage diabetics. *Acta Paediatr Scand (Suppl)* 1980; **283**: 50–52.
13. Hillson RM. Diabetes outward bound mountain course, Eskdale, Cumbria. *Diab Med* 1985; **2**: 217–224.
14. Newton RW, Isles T, Farquhar JW. The Firbush Project – sharing a way of life. *Diab Med* 1985; **2**: 217–224.
15. Semiz S, Bilgin UO, Bundak R, Bircan I. Summer camps for diabetic children: an experience in Antalya, Turkey. *Acta Diabetol* 2000; **37**: 197–200.
16. Misuraca A, DiGennaro M, Lioniello M *et al.* Summer camps for diabetic children: an experience in Campania, Italy. *Diabet Res Clin Pract* 1996; **32**: 91–96.

17. American Diabetes Association. Management of diabetes at diabetes camps. *Diabetes Care* 2001; **S1**: S113–S115.
18. Dublon V, Morjaria A. Children's diabetic camps: doctors can gain too. *Br Med J* 2003; **21**: 326.
19. American Diabetes Association. *Camp Implementation Guide*. Alexandria, VA: American Diabetes Association, 1999.
20. Frost GF, Hodges S, Swift PGF. Dietary carbohydrate deficits and hypoglycaemia in the young diabetic on holiday. *Diab Med* 1986; **3**: 250–252.
21. Swift PGF, Waldon S. Have diabetes – will travel. *Pract Diabet* 1990; **7**: 101–104.
22. Braatveldt GD, Midenhall L, Patten C, Harris G. Insulin requirements and metabolic control in children with diabetes mellitus attending a summer camp. *Diab Med* 1997; **14**: 258–261.
23. Gale E, Bennet T, Green GH, MacDonald I. Hypoglycaemia, hypothermia and shivering in man. *Diabetes Care* 1987; **10**: 584–588.
24. MacDonald MJ. Post-exercise late-onset hypoglycaemia in insulin-dependent diabetic patients. *Diabetes Care* 1987; **10**: 584–588.
25. Wahren J, Felig P, Ahlborg G, Jorfeldt L. Glucose metabolism during leg exercise in man. *J Clin Invest* 1971; **50**: 2712–2725.
26. Davis SN, Mann S, Galassetti P *et al.* Effects of differing durations of antecedent hypoglycaemia on counterregulatory responses to subsequent hypoglycaemia in normal humans. *Diabetes* 2000; **49**: 1897–1093.
27. Dandona P, Hooke D, Bell J. Exercise and insulin absorption from subcutaneous tissue. *Br Med J* 1978; **1**: 479–481.
28. Koivisto VA, Felig P. Effects of leg exercise on insulin absorption in diabetic patients. *New Engl J Med* 1978; **298**: 79–83.
29. Kemmer FW, Berchtold P, Berger M *et al.* Exercise induced fall in blood glucose concentration is unrelated to alteration of insulin metabolism. *Diabetes* 1979; **28**: 1131–1137.

8
Insulin Pump Therapy and Exercise

Peter Hammond and **Sandra Dudley**

8.1 Introduction

Continuous subcutaneous insulin infusion (CSII) is a method of insulin delivery, in which a small pager-sized, portable, programmable pump infuses insulin from a reservoir of short-acting or rapid-acting analogue insulin, through a catheter attached to a cannula whose tip is placed subcutaneously, usually in the anterior abdominal wall (Figure 8.1). The pump can deliver insulin at variable hourly infusion rates through the day (basal insulin), and insulin boluses can be administered at mealtimes, according to the carbohydrate intake of the meal. In this way CSII is able to achieve circulating insulin levels which more closely approximate the normal physiological state in non-diabetic subjects than other conventional methods of insulin administration. Use of CSII can have particular advantages for maintaining more even glycaemic control both during and after exercise.

8.2 Potential Advantages of CSII

Small volumes of insulin are infused every few minutes using CSII, which means that there is virtually no insulin depot in the subcutaneous tissue at the infusion site. Consequently there is a much more predictable relationship between insulin delivery and circulating insulin levels. The day-to-day variation in circulating insulin for an individual using CSII is less than 2 per cent, compared with a variation ranging from 10 to 50 per cent for those using short-acting and intermediate-acting insulin.[1]

Exercise and Sport in Diabetes, 2nd Edition   Edited by Dinesh Nagi
© 2005 John Wiley & Sons, Ltd.

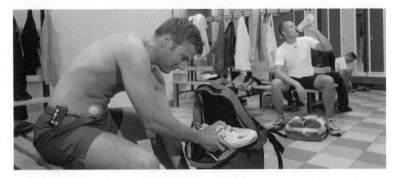

Figure 8.1 Medtronic insulin infusion pump in position on an athlete's abdominal wall. Reproduced by permission of Medtronic.com

Advances in pump technology allow the basal rate of infusion to be varied hour to hour, so that insulin delivery is very well matched to patient needs. This results in consistently lower hypoglycaemia rates in studies comparing CSII with intensified insulin regimens using multiple daily injections.[2]

Using the latest pumps, bolus doses of insulin can be matched not only to carbohydrate intake, but the type of meal can be taken into account. Meals resulting in prolonged carbohydrate absorption, such as pizza or Chinese food, can be matched with a prolonged (square-wave) insulin bolus or a dual peak and square-wave bolus, rather than the normal bolus peak. Additional insulin boli can also be given if a pump user has a significant snack, or if an error in calculating a bolus dose results in a higher than expected blood glucose level (correction bolus). In this way, use of CSII not only reduces the incidence of hypoglycaemia for the same levels of blood glucose control, but also reduces the fluctuations in blood glucose levels which are the norm for those using multiple injections. CSII users often report that they recognize blood glucose levels above $10\,\text{mmol}\,\text{l}^{-1}$, from symptoms such as fatigue, nausea and headache, in contrast to those using multiple injections, who usually only notice symptoms at much higher levels, because frequent levels above $10\,\text{mmol}\,\text{l}^{-1}$ are commonplace with such a regimen.

These reductions in blood glucose fluctuation result in an improved quality of life for those switching from multiple injections to CSII. They report a greater sense of well-being, greater exercise capacity, more lifestyle flexibility, particularly with regard to diet and travel, and less diabetes-related worry.[2]

8.3 CSII Usage

International usage of CSII is highly variable, largely as a result of the cost, which is approximately £1000 per patient per year. This includes the cost of the pump itself, averaged over 4 years, and the annual cost of consumables. In the USA it is estimated that 20 per cent of those with type 1 diabetes are on insulin pumps. This may reflect the fact that about two-thirds of American physicians with type 1 diabetes use a pump – or that Miss America 1998 has very publicly used and promoted CSII! In Europe, Germany has the highest reported rate of pump usage, with an estimated 15 per cent of those with type 1 diabetes. Most other Western European countries have estimated usage rates of 5–10 per cent and usage is increasing in many Eastern European countries. In the UK CSII usage has been very low and even now it is probably only used by around 1 per cent of those with type 1 diabetes. NICE (the National Institute for Clinical Excellence) published guidance on the use of CSII in 2003, recommending that CSII should be made available to those with type 1 diabetes who fail to achieve their blood glucose control target because of disabling hypoglycaemia on multiple daily injection regimens.[3]

8.4 Benefits of CSII Over Multiple Daily Injections

Many of the studies comparing CSII with multiple daily injections were performed using the original basic pumps, which had a fixed basal insulin infusion rate and were much less reliable than modern pumps. Despite this, meta-analyses which include these initial studies still show benefit in terms of small improvements in blood glucose control, and significant reductions in hypoglycaemia and fluctuation in blood glucose levels.[2,4] In the Diabetes Control and Complications Trial (DCCT), CSII was an option in the intensive treatment arm. Some 42 per cent of those in this arm were using CSII rather than multiple injections at the study end. Those using CSII for most of the study showed improved blood glucose control compared with those using mostly multiple daily injections.[5] Improvements in blood glucose control with CSII are most pronounced for those using carbohydrate counting to match bolus doses to food intake and monitoring blood glucose levels frequently, with at least four estimations each day.[6]

Recent studies using rapid-acting analogue insulin in the pumps have shown that these give superior glycaemic control to both CSII using conventional short-acting insulins and to multiple daily injections with rapid-acting insulin analogues.[7] There have been no large studies comparing CSII with multiple injection regimens using long-acting insulin analogues, such as glargine, but preliminary evidence suggests potential benefits for CSII for various parameters of glycaemic control.[8] There is also increasing evidence that the benefits of CSII extend to children and adolescents.[9]

There is much qualitative information about the impact of CSII on quality of life, but objective evidence is limited. Adolescents opting to use pump therapy rather than multiple injections demonstrated improvements in coping ability.[9] In a crossover trial comparing CSII with multiple daily injections, subjects reported improved quality of life in a number of areas, most notably daily activities, eating and sleeping.[10]

The benefits of CSII are seen principally in people with type 1 diabetes, with recent studies failing to show convincing benefit in those with type 2 diabetes,[11] and the following discussion of its advantages in the context of exercise will be limited to those with type 1 diabetes.

8.5 Potential Advantages for CSII Use with Exercise

The person using any subcutaneous insulin injection regimen is likely to have a significant insulin depot when they take exercise, produced by a combination of short- and intermediate-acting insulin or analogue insulin – even if they have made allowance for exercise by reducing their usual insulin dosage. CSII results in a much smaller subcutaneous insulin depot, probably an order of magnitude less than that produced by subcutaneous injection regimens. The advantage for the pump user taking exercise is that circulating free insulin levels are lower than for the injection user, both during and after exercise. Furthermore a smaller insulin depot means circulating levels are less subject to an increase in absorption from exercise-induced changes in blood flow. Lower circulating free insulin levels have two consequences: a reduced risk of hypoglycaemia, and improved fuel mobilization, particularly from breakdown of liver glycogen, which is inhibited by the higher circulating levels in those using subcutaneous injections. The pump user can also be more spontaneous about exercise, as an adjustment to the basal rate will effectively reduce free circulating insulin levels within an hour to protect against hypoglycaemia, whereas the injection user can do nothing about the insulin already injected. In this way the pump user can have a metabolic response to exercise that approximates to normal.

8.6 Studies of Response to Exercise in CSII Users

Studies comparing the effect of CSII vs injection regimens on the response to exercise mostly date from the early 1980s when the pump technology was less sophisticated, with fixed basal infusion rates and a single bolus facility, and short-acting soluble insulin was infused rather than rapid-acting analogue insulin. Despite this, many of the theoretical advantages of CSII over injection regimens were confirmed. All the studies investigated subjects with type 1 diabetes.

The benefits in terms of circulating free insulin levels were shown by Viberti et al.,[12] who studied eight subjects initially using a mixture of short and intermediate-acting insulin two or three times a day, then using CSII, which was started 3 weeks prior to the test. They performed moderately intense exercise 2 h after breakfast. Whilst using injections blood glucose levels were higher at the start of exercise, around $12\,\text{mmol}\,\text{l}^{-1}$, falling by over $7.5\,\text{mmol}\,\text{l}^{-1}$, compared with a starting glucose of about $7\,\text{mmol}\,\text{l}^{-1}$ and a fall of $3.5\,\text{mmol}\,\text{l}^{-1}$ when using the pump. There was no increase in circulating free insulin levels whilst using CSII, compared with a significant rise whilst on the injection regimen. This rise was accompanied by an increased growth hormone response.

It is important to remember that, whilst exercise does not increase free insulin levels in the pump user, the improved efficacy of absorption with CSII means that free insulin levels will rise more rapidly after a bolus than with a short-acting injection. Thus, when exercising soon after a meal, the pump user may experience hypoglycaemia if the bolus dose is not adjusted. This was demonstrated by Koivisto, who found that blood glucose levels fell 60 per cent more in pump users exercising 90 min after breakfast than in those on a conventional subcutaneous insulin regimen.[13]

It is also of note that a short burst of strenuous activity may result in hyperglycaemia. Mitchell studied eight CSII users with type 1 diabetes who performed a short period of exercise at 80 per cent VO_{2max} in the post-absorptive state.[14] When subjects were initially normoglycaemic, blood glucose levels increased by a mean of 2.3 mmol l^{-1}. This was sustained for about 2 h post-exercise.

8.7   Practicalities for Using CSII with Exercise

Just as with those individuals using subcutaneous insulin injection regimens, there are no hard and fast rules about the adjustments needed when exercising. Each person will need to monitor blood glucose levels closely when starting any new exercise, assessing the immediate effects and the longer-term potential for hypoglycaemia as muscle glycogen stores are replenished. In this way the appropriate adjustments to the pump regimen can be made.

Those who habitually take exercise on a pump often find that only minor adjustments are needed to their regimen once a training programme is established as the variations in their regimen have been built-in to their usual routine. However, those who exercise on a more occasional basis usually have to make more significant alterations.

Two techniques are available to the pump user for managing glucose levels when taking exercise – pump-on or pump-off.[15] It is preferable to use the pump-on approach whenever possible as this will optimize fuel utilization for exercise. However there are certain situations where the pump-on approach is either contraindicated to some extent (see below), or where individual preference is for the pump-off technique.

Pump-on

The adjustment to the insulin regimen with the pump-on approach will depend on a number of factors: the nature of the exercise, its duration, the timing of exercise in relation to meals and the degree of planning. It is possible, of course, to allow for the effect of exercise on blood glucose levels by increasing carbohydrate consumption. However this is not as necessary for the pump user who, by reducing the insulin infusion rate, can facilitate mobilization of fuel from carbohydrate and fat metabolism to compensate for the associated energy consumption.

If exercise is taking place within 2–3 h of a meal then the bolus dose before that meal should be reduced. The reduction will depend on the intensity and duration of the exercise. For example mild exertion, such as a gentle walk, lasting for about an hour might require a 15 per cent reduction in the insulin bolus, whilst strenuous exertion, such as mountain biking, lasting for 3 h, might need as much as a 50 per cent decrease. More prolonged and more strenuous exertion is more likely to result in hypoglycaemia, both immediately after the exercise and delayed as a result of muscle re-filling. Thus, with this sort of exercise, reductions in the basal rate are also required. These reductions will usually be similar to the reductions in bolus doses and the duration of the reduction may need to be for several hours. Again, individual monitoring is the key to successful management.

Basal rate reduction should be used either in combination with bolus dose reductions as above, or if exercise takes place more than 3–4 h post-prandially. The simplest approach is to initially reduce all basal rates by 50 per cent during activity and gauge future adjustments according to how well blood glucose levels are maintained immediately after exertion. If basal rates are reduced then ideally this should commence, for those using rapid acting analogues, at least 60 min before circulating insulin levels need to fall, to minimize the risk of hypoglycaemia. This is obviously possible when exercise is planned well in advance, but this will not be the case for more spontaneous activity and so additional corrections may need to be made in this situation, usually in the form of increased carbohydrate intake. After exercise basal rates will need to be reduced as for post-prandial exertion and additionally the next bolus dose should be decreased to minimize the risk of delayed hypoglycaemia.

The only time when the insulin regimen may not need to be altered is when strenuous exercise is performed for a short period of time, probably less than 15 min. In this situation blood glucose levels may rise and so insulin doses should not be reduced in advance.

Ideally the pump user will achieve an appropriate balance of basal and bolus insulin adjustment and extra carbohydrate intake to get optimal glycaemic control, fuel utilization and weight reduction. There are charts that give an estimate of the likely calorie consumption associated with various forms of exercise according to an individual's weight,[16] or alternatively calorie counters can be used whilst exercising. In this way the amount of carbohydrate equating to the calories used can be estimated. This can be made up by any combination of extra carbohydrate intake and reduced insulin doses. The pump user should know their insulin–carbohydrate ratio and hence be able to make a reasonable prediction for the change in insulin dose required. For example if the exercise consumes the equivalent of 64 calories of carbohydrate and the insulin–carbohydrate ratio is usually 1:8 (one unit of insulin is required per 8 g carbohydrate to maintain the same blood glucose level), then a reduction in insulin dose of 8 units will be needed, or a reduction of 4 units and consumption of an extra 32 g carbohydrate.

If weight reduction through exercise is an important goal then the temptation will be to rely solely on insulin dose reduction to manage exercise. This may be acceptable, but insulin doses should not be reduced by more than 50 per cent or control of fuel metabolism may become uncontrolled, and the risk of ketoacidosis starts to rise.[16]

Pump-off

Unsurprisingly, this approach to managing exercise involves removing the pump during physical activity. This is not usually the preferred option for the reasons mentioned above. If there is a need or desire to remove the pump during exercise then consideration needs to be given to the best way of providing adequate circulating insulin levels during activity. Removal of the pump for 1–2 h is usually not a problem for rapid-acting analogue users, and ideally the physical activity will be sufficiently strenuous to maintain controlled blood glucose levels. If this is not the case, or activity is more prolonged, then it may be necessary to temporarily increase the basal rate in the lead-up to the activity. A bolus of insulin, either via the pump or an injection, can be administered prior to starting the exercise, but the rapid onset of action will significantly increase the risk of hypoglycaemia. If this approach is used, a reasonable initial bolus would be 50 per cent of the total basal infusion that would normally be administered over the period during which activity is being taken. Once the activity has stopped and the pump is running again, the same adjustments will be needed to the basal rate as for the pump-on option to reduce the risk of immediate or delayed hypoglycaemia.

8.8   Cautions for Using CSII with Exercise

There are a few pitfalls which need to be considered when pump users take exercise, in particular related to contact sports, water sports and winter sports.[17] Pump users need to take care to avoid displacement of the infusion set during exercise as the onset of ketoacidosis can occur within 5 h of cessation of infusion of a rapid-acting analogue insulin. The pump user must check that the infusion set is still intact on a regular basis, and frequent blood glucose monitoring will help identify any infusion problem. This is particularly an issue with excessive sweating and with contact sports.

Sweating is a universal accompaniment of significant physical activity and may prove problematic for fixing the insulin infusion set. Strategies for avoiding problems with fixation are use of an antiperspirant around, but not onto, the infusion site; or application of strong adhesives to increase the adhesion of the infusion set. Liquid skin preparations can be particularly helpful to improve fixation.

Contact sports, such as rugby or basketball, predispose the pump user to pump displacement, and the individual may feel more comfortable with using a pump-off strategy whilst engaged in these sports. Alternatively a protective case can be used to minimize the risk of damage to the pump.

Some pumps are allegedly waterproof, but it is prudent to either keep the pump in a waterproof case or remove it completely during exercise involving water. The latter approach is particularly advisable where the water sport is more vigorous, such as water polo or surfing.

Temperature extremes cause insulin degradation and this is most relevant with respect to winter sports. In order to keep the insulin infusion at an adequate ambient temperature the pump should be worn inside an inner layer of clothing.

Traction on the infusion set during exercise may cause irritation at the infusion site. This can be reduced by using flexible Teflon infusion sets. Similarly, those using pump-off strategies for exercise may prefer to use quick release infusion sets which allow disconnection and reconnection without having to resite the infusion set.

In conclusion taking exercise for the person with type 1 diabetes can be made significantly easier by using an insulin pump. Fluctuations in blood glucose levels can be reduced by optimal use of the pump. Pump users may initially be concerned about potential damage to the pump or infusion set during exertion but can be reassured that this is extremely unlikely during most activities.

References

1. Lauritzen T, Pramming S, Deckert T, Binder C. Pharmacokinetics of continuous subcutaneous insulin infusion. *Diabetologia* 1983; **24**: 326–329.
2. Lenhard MJ, Reeves GD. Continuous subcutaneous insulin infusion: a comprehensive review of insulin pump therapy. *Arch Intern Med* 2001; **161**: 2293–2300.
3. NICE Technology Appraisal no. 57: Diabetes (type 1) – insulin pump therapy, 2003.
4. Pickup J, Mattock M, Kerry S. Glycaemic control with continuous subcutaneous insulin infusion compared with intensive insulin injections in patients with type 1 diabetes: meta-analysis of randomised controlled trials. *Br Med J* 2002; **324**: 1–6.
5. The Diabetes Control and Complications Trial Research Group. The effect of intensive treatment of diabetes on the development and progression of long-term complications in insulin-dependent diabetes. *New Engl J Med* 1993; **329**: 977–986.
6. Bode B, Steed D, Davidson P. Determinants of glycemic control in insulin pump therapy. *Diabetes* 1997; 46 (suppl. 1): **143**.
7. Hanaire-Broutin H, Melki V, Bessieres-Lacombe S, Tauber J-P. Comparison of continuous subcutaneous insulin infusion and multiple daily injection regimens using insulin lispro in type 1 diabetic patients on intensified insulin. *Diabetes Care* 2000; **23**: 1232–1235.

8. Doyle EA, Weinzimer SA, Steffen AT, Ahern JH, Vincent M, Tamborlane WV. A randomized, prospective trial comparing the efficacy of continuous subcutaneous insulin infusion with multiple daily injections using insulin glargine. *Diabetes Care* 2004; **27**: 1554–1558.

9. Boland EA, Grey M, Oesterle A, Fredrickson L, Tamborlane WY. Continuous subcutaneous insulin infusion. A new way to lower risk of severe hypoglycaemia, improve metabolic control, and enhance coping in adolescents with type 1 diabetes. *Diabetes Care* 1999; **22**: 1779–1784.

10. Hammond PJ, Kerr D, Everett J, Dudley S. Randomised controlled comparison of CSII (continuous subcutaneous insulin infusion) and multiple daily injections (MDI) on glycaemic control and quality of life during intensive treatment of type 1 diabetes. UK experience within the 5-Nations study. *Diab Med* 2004; **21**(s2).

11. Raskin P, Bode BW, Marks JB, Hirsch IB, Weinstein RL, McGill JB, Peterson GE, Mudaliar SR, Reinhardt RR. Continuous subcutaneous insulin infusion and multiple daily injection therapy are equally effective in type 2 diabetes: a randomized, parallel-group, 24-week study. *Diabetes Care* 2003; **26**: 2598–2603.

12. Viberti GC, Home PD, Bilous RW, Alberti KGMM, Dalton N, Keen H, Pickup JC. Metabolic effects on physical exercise in insulin-dependent diabetics controlled by subcutaneous insulin infusion on conventional injection therapy. *Acta Endocrinol (Copenh)* 1984; **105**: 515–520.

13. Koivisto VA, Tronier B. Postprandial blood glucose response to exercise in type 1 diabetes: comparison between pump and injection therapy. *Diabetes Care* 1983; **6**: 436–440.

14. Mitchell TH, Abraham G, Schiffrin A, Leiter LA, Marliss EB. Hyperglycaemia after intense exercise in IDDM subjects during continuous subcutaneous insulin infusion. *Diabetes Care* 1988; **11**: 311–317.

15. Zinman B. Exercise and the pump. In *The Insulin Pump Therapy Book*. Minimed Technologies: Sylmar, CA, 1995; 106–115.

16. Walsh J, Roberts R. ExCarbs for exercise. In *Pumping Insulin*. Torrey Pines Press: San Diego, CA, 2000; 169–180.

17. Colberg SR, Walsh PA. Pumping insulin during exercise. *Physician Sports Med* 2002; **30**: 33–38.

9
Diabetes and the Marathon

Bill Burr

9.1 Introduction

The marathon represents a supreme athletic challenge, and for those runners who also happen to have diabetes the challenge is even more daunting. An individual with diabetes who is contemplating running a marathon should be fairly clear about the magnitude of the undertaking, and their reasons for attempting it. The extreme nature of the exertion and the sustained training required over many months demand enormous attention to detail, and will almost certainly cause problems with diabetic control.

There are many variables affecting diabetic control in relation to marathon running, and it is difficult to produce a single set of recommendations. People vary in physique and level of fitness as well as in athletic ability. On top of this, people with diabetes have additional variables related to such things as their treatment regimen and insulin type and dosage. They also vary in terms of the speed with which they become hyperglycaemic and develop ketones when insulin levels are inadequate. If an individual has absolutely no ability to secrete insulin, their insulin requirement is about 1 unit kg^{-1} body weight day^{-1}. They will tend to become hyperglycaemic quite rapidly when insulin-deprived. People with lower insulin requirements have varying degrees of residual insulin secretion, and tend to be less prone to severe hyperglycaemia and ketosis. It may be somewhat easier for such an individual to maintain metabolic control during the severe physical stresses of the marathon than for someone with no residual insulin secretion. It follows that there will inevitably be a great deal of trial and error before a particular individual discovers the precise adjustments to their diabetic routine

Exercise and Sport in Diabetes, 2nd Edition   Edited by Dinesh Nagi
© 2005 John Wiley & Sons, Ltd.

which will enable them to train and compete safely and effectively in the marathon.

Some general guidelines will be given, and then a number of examples of how different individuals have put these into practice.

9.2   Guidelines

Pre-exercise health check

If you have not been in the habit of taking regular exercise, it would be wise to consult your general practitioner or hospital consultant to make sure there are no health reasons why you should avoid heavy exertion. The examination should include feet, eyes, heart and chest, and measurement of blood pressure. The urine should be checked for protein, and glycated haemoglobin (HbAlc) should be measured to check diabetic control. Depending on age and/or symptoms, it may be considered advisable to have an ECG or exercise test.

Footwear, clothing and equipment

Clothing should be comfortable; shorts need to have a pocket for dextrose tablets. A tracksuit is needed for cold weather only. Shoes are the most important item of equipment, especially for runs over about 4 miles. They need to be good quality, well fitting and must be 'broken-in' carefully during shorter runs, with a special check of the feet for any signs of blistering. They need thick, shock-absorbing soles, and in addition it is sensible to wear hosiery which has maximum cushioning ability (e.g. Thorlo). When training, or even when competing, it may be useful to carry a 'bumbag' or small rucksack containing blood testing kit, identification, glucose tablets and drinks, contact numbers and advice for dealing with hypoglycaemia.

Keeping in contact

It is wise to make sure that someone knows where you are going to be running, and what time you expect to return. This is important on dark evenings and on little-used roads, and is absolutely essential when running cross-country. However well prepared you are, there is going to be an increased risk of hypoglycaemia when running, and it is vital that help should be available when this happens. It is also important to wear some form of identification, such as an 'SOS' bracelet, to confirm the fact that you have diabetes and to give a contact number in case of emergency.

It is worth giving some thought to the idea of joining a local running club. This can provide a source of running partners, as well as providing advice on type and availability of equipment, and on loosening-up exercises.

Diary

Mention has already been made of the trial-and-error approach which is needed while tailoring diet and insulin regimen to suit different training and competition schedules. The learning process is greatly helped if detailed records are kept – especially in the early stages. Ideally a log-book should contain details of:

- distance run;

- time taken;

- blood glucose levels before and after run;

- timing, amount, and type of insulin before and after;

- timing, amount, and type of food taken 2–3 h before and up to 8 h after the run;

- time of day;

- weather conditions and an estimate of the effect these have on the intensity of effort;

- hypoglycaemia – timing, warning symptoms (e.g. weakness, blurred vision, feeling dizzy or maybe no warning), action taken;

- general comments, e.g. hypoglycaemia occurring 12 h afterwards, or overnight, changes in fitness and running speed, changes in body weight (lower body weight will reduce insulin requirements) and ideas for future treatment adjustments.

Training

The golden rule is to build up gradually both the length and the intensity of training runs. Where you actually start from will depend on your general level of fitness, and on whether or not you are running or taking part in active sports on a regular basis. For instance, a sedentary, inactive person should begin by walking, and build up both speed and distance (e.g. $\frac{1}{2}$, 1, 2, 3 miles) before starting to jog. If you are regularly playing sport such as soccer, rugby or squash you will probably be able to start by jogging 2–3 miles, and build up from this.

As the person with diabetes starts to do endurance training on a regular basis (say three training runs per week), there will be a progressive reduction in insulin requirements of between 25 and 40 per cent. This is irrespective of any insulin reductions needed on the day of exercise, and is a reflection of the improved insulin sensitivity brought about by regular exercise. Most athletes find that this insulin sensitivity wears off within about a week when training stops.

Diabetic control and monitoring

The need for good diabetic control before exercise has been stressed before (see Chapter 2). Ideally, the blood glucose should be between 6 and 10 mmol l^{-1} (110–180 mg dl^{-1}) at the start of exertion. If the glucose is above 14 mmol l^{-1} (250 mg dl^{-1}), the urine should be checked for ketones, and if they are present the session should be cancelled. Figure 9.1 shows how exercise can cause serious worsening of ketosis in an individual whose diabetes is out of control at the start of exercise.

As mentioned elsewhere, the physiological response in a non-diabetic to endurance events is to reduce insulin levels to a minimum, to allow release of glucose from the liver, and to make sure that glucose uptake by muscles is not excessive. The person with diabetes has to try to mimic this situation by reducing insulin doses, but without becoming deficient in insulin to the point of allowing ketoacidosis to occur.

Blood glucose will need to be checked 15–30 min before training or competing, as mentioned above. If it is below 6 mmol l^{-1}, extra carbohydrate in the form of a chocolate bar or high-carbohydrate drink is needed. Some athletes have recommended testing blood glucose hourly throughout the marathon, but this would seem excessive for most people, and is perhaps feasible only during training runs.

After running, it is necessary to check blood glucose after 30 min or so, to guide the amount of carbohydrate replacement required. Monitoring can revert to normal after this, with the exception that it is absolutely vital to check blood glucose before bed to try to avoid overnight hypoglycaemia.

Insulin dose

It is really difficult to generalize about the extent of insulin dose reductions for the marathon. The simplest situation is that of someone on treatment with a continuous subcutaneous insulin infusion. These people find that the basal infusion rate needs to be reduced by 50 per cent or more, and additional carbohydrate may still have to be taken during the event. For people on treatment with infused soluble insulin (e.g. Actrapid or Humulin S), the infusion rate needs to be reduced 30 min *before*

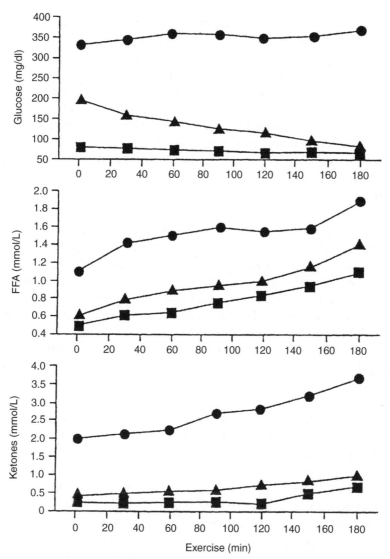

Figure 9.1 Effect of prolonged exercise on blood glucose, plasma ketone bodies (acetoacetate and β-hydroxybutyrate) and plasma free fatty acids (FFA) in healthy control participants (■), diabetic patients in moderate control (▲) and ketotic diabetic patients (●). Adapted from Berger M *et al.*, *Diabetologia* 1977; **13**: 355–365 by permission

the race. If the insulin analogue Humalog (lispro insulin) is being infused, the rate can be reduced immediately before the event because of the rapid absorption of subcutaneous Humalog.

The most common insulin regimen in Europe is the so-called 'basal/bolus' regimen, in which a bedtime dose of isophane, lente or ultralente insulin is taken together with pre-prandial soluble insulin or Humalog. On this type of treatment schedule, most athletes would take the normal dose of insulin on the night before the marathon, or would make only a slight reduction (10 per cent). They would make variable and, at times, radical reductions in the preprandial dose before the event. The range of dose reduction ranges from about 20 to 90 per cent, and one of the major factors determining the size of the reduction is the amount of planned carbohydrate intake during the race (see below). The timing of the soluble insulin injection before a race is critical. It is important that the insulin levels are declining before starting sustained exercise, and this means that the injection of soluble insulin should be about 90–120 min before the race, while Humalog should be taken about 60 min before the event.

One other insulin regimen which is still quite commonly encountered is that in which there is a twice-daily injection of a mixture of soluble and isophane or lente insulins. It is probably better for an athlete to be using free mixtures of short- and intermediate-acting insulins rather than pre-mixed insulins, since this allows a greater degree of flexibility in adjusting doses to cope with training and competitions. For races taking place in the morning, the reductions in short-acting insulin would be similar to those made on a basal/bolus regimen, together with a modest reduction in intermediate insulin (about 20 per cent). For races in the afternoon, the morning short-acting insulin would not be altered, but the intermediate insulin would be drastically reduced or omitted.

After the race, people again have differing approaches to making adjustments to their insulin dose. Many athletes take quite large amounts of freely absorbed carbohydrate 30–60 min after the race, and if so they would take either the usual insulin to cover this or would make a modest reduction. Later in the day and overnight, and even through the next day, there is going to be a strong tendency to develop delayed hypoglycaemia, which has to be countered by extra carbohydrate intake and reduced insulin. The reasons for this have been explained elsewhere (Chapter 2) but, in simple terms, sustained exercise has a dramatic and prolonged (12–24 h or more) effect on muscle sensitivity to insulin. More glucose is removed from the bloodstream for a given amount of insulin. Muscle glycogen stores are being replenished during this time, and this increases the demand for blood glucose (Chapter 1). It is reasonable to reduce the bedtime insulin on a basal/bolus regimen by 20 per cent or so, and to make a similar reduction to the teatime intermediate insulin for those on twice-daily injections, and to combine this with a substantial increase in evening carbohydrate intake.

Food and fluid intake

General dietary guidelines for those taking part in demanding athletic events, involving sustained, high-intensity effort, are summarized in Table 9.1. Advice specifically relating to the marathon is given below.

Table 9.1 Summary of dietary recommendations for elite athletes

Four days before competition

- Taper training
- Carbohydrate loading: 8–10 g kg^{-1} body mass per day for 3–4 days

Before competition

- 3–4 h before competition, eat easily digestible high carbohydrate meal, 1–2 g kg^{-1} body mass
- For competitors who have diabetes, this meal should consist of carbohydrates with a low glycaemic index
- Avoid concentrated (>8 % glucose) glucose drinks within 1 h of exercise (risk of gastrointestinal discomfort)

During exercise

- Carbohydrate–electrolyte solutions are helpful and delay glycogen depletion and avoid dehydration
- Suitable sports drinks should be consumed at the rate of 120–150 ml for every 15 min exercise

During recovery from exercise

- 50 g carbohydrate immediately after exercise and 8–10 g carbohydrate kg^{-1} body weight in 24 h. High-glycaemic-index foods in the first 6 h, and continued for the 24 h when rapid recovery is needed
- Athletes with diabetes should avoid high-glycaemic-index foods, except in the immediate post-exercise period
- Addition of protein may speed recovery of glycogen stores

Several days pre-event

Before undertaking a major endurance event such as the marathon, it is customary to phase-down training in the week before the event, and to increase carbohydrate intake to 70 per cent or more of the calorie intake. For those with diabetes, this advice would seem to hold true, but for the purposes of so-called 'carbo-loading', it would be wise to stick to foods with a low glycaemic index (see Chapter 1). These carbohydrate foods are complex, require digestion to take place before absorption of simple sugars can occur, and therefore have the least effect on blood glucose and insulin requirements. The recommended daily intake of carbohydrate for those who do not have diabetes is 8–10 g kg^{-1} body weight for 3 or 4 days before the race, and there is no reason why this advice should not apply also for those with diabetes.

Pre-exercise meals

Most people with diabetes feel that it is important to have a substantial, high-carbohydrate meal before the competition. This advice has been summed up as 'it's important to have ballast in the hold'. The drawback is that many people feel uncomfortable or are prone to stomach cramps if they eat excessively before exercise. As a compromise, the pre-marathon meal should be taken about 2 h before the event for those using ordinary soluble insulin. For those using Humalog, 1–1.5 h before the race would be appropriate. For this meal, it would be sensible to use mainly carbohydrate with a low glycaemic index. The amount to be taken will be governed by trial and error, according to the amount that can comfortably be eaten. As a guide, it would be reasonable to aim for 2–4 g carbohydrate per kg body weight.

Pre-exercise drinks

As mentioned in Chapter 1, ingestion of high-carbohydrate (25 per cent or more) drinks before a race is not recommended because of the tendency to cause delayed stomach emptying and gastrointestinal disturbance. Commercially available carbohydrate–electrolyte solutions contain 5–8 per cent carbohydrate, and do not cause delayed stomach emptying or abdominal cramps. It is reasonable to use these immediately before the race, especially if there is a need to correct relative hypoglycaemia at this time (blood glucose <6 mmol l^{-1}). It should be possible to drink 500 ml of these solutions without detriment to athletic performance.

Carbohydrate intake during the race

It is important to take regular fluid throughout the race to prevent dehydration, and this fluid should be taken regularly according to a fixed plan, without waiting for the development of thirst. Carbohydrate–electrolyte drinks have been developed commercially for just this type of situation, and have been found to be well tolerated. Chapter 1 summed up evidence to show that taking these solutions regularly through prolonged exercise has a glycogen-sparing action which delays the onset of exhaustion. People with diabetes may also benefit from taking these drinks, although it will be necessary to experiment during long-distance training runs to discover how much can be taken without producing hyperglycaemia. The prevailing levels of blood insulin will be a major determining factor, but it is also true that actively contracting muscles are remarkably able to dispose of blood glucose in the presence of very low levels of insulin.

If you have successfully reduced your insulin you may have no need to take additional carbohydrate during the race, and many athletes with diabetes prefer to run the whole distance with virtually no additional carbohydrate. Others prefer to take additional food in the form of bananas, cereal bars or chocolate.

Carbohydrate and food intake after exercise

Very rapid recovery from exercise is only strictly relevant to athletes who are taking part in events which require daily performance for days or weeks. There is evidence that restoration of muscle glycogen levels and exercise capacity can be speeded by taking high-glycaemic-index carbohydrates, and by increasing daily carbohydrate intake by 50 per cent (from 6 to 9 g kg^{-1} body weight per day). For the 'ordinary' marathon runner with diabetes, it is probably sufficient to replace carbohydrate and fluid immediately after the event using carbohydrate–electrolyte solutions. Later in the day it would be wise to take a large meal consisting mainly of low-glycaemic-index carbohydrate to assist the replenishment of glycogen stores overnight. Even with reductions of insulin dose and extra carbohydrate, there will still be a tendency to hypoglycaemia on the following morning, requiring extra carbohydrate and reduced insulin. Some athletes report that this effect can continue for 48 h.

9.3   Personal Views

Dawn Kenwright

Dawn was already an international athlete when she developed type 1 diabetes in 1993, at the age of 37. She specialized in mountain and cross-country running. She was hospitalized to commence insulin treatment, but started running again within 3 days of discharge, actually competed 3 weeks after this, and ran in an international after 6 weeks!

She attributes her success to great determination and discipline in taking four injections of insulin daily and monitoring and recording blood sugars regularly, as well as controlling diet and mealtimes. She runs a lot on her own, and stresses the need to carry identification, to let people know of her whereabouts, and to carry adequate supplies of glucose.

Dawn's insulin regimen consists of human soluble insulin 4, 4 and 6 units before breakfast, lunch and evening meal, respectively, and 8 units of human isophane at night. She monitors blood glucose before and after every run, and sometimes during runs when not competing. She reduces her soluble insulin before major events, and takes large amounts of complex carbohydrate during the build-up. During an event, she finds that she is unable to eat carbohydrate, and she also cannot tolerate isotonic drinks. She has managed to run for 5 h at high altitude without taking carbohydrate. She takes complex carbohydrate soon after the run, and has a marked tendency to delayed hypoglycaemia 24 or even 48 h after the event.

Matthew Kiln

Dr Matthew Kiln is a general practitioner who has run more than 12 marathons. He has type 1 diabetes, which is controlled by twice-daily injections of a mixture of soluble and lente insulins. He uses beef insulins, having experienced problems with hypoglycaemia while taking human insulin.

During training runs of up to 15 miles, Matthew prefers to take his usual insulin dose while maintaining his blood glucose with frequent carbohydrates. At times he has found difficulties in taking adequate carbohydrate without feeling sick, because by trial and error he has established that he needs about 7–12 g of carbohydrate per mile. This varies according to the time of day, and is presumably related to the level of free insulin circulating during the run.

For the marathon itself Matthew switches his approach, and takes a drastically reduced dose of soluble insulin only on the morning of the race, taking for instance just 2 units of soluble insulin instead of his usual 4 units soluble and 14 units lente. With this low dose, and taking 30 g of carbohydrate during the race, he began with a blood sugar of $7 \, \text{mmol} \, \text{l}^{-1}$, and finished with a blood glucose of $4 \, \text{mmol} \, \text{l}^{-1}$.

9.4 Summary

Even though running the marathon is a supreme athletic challenge, many people with diabetes have successfully attempted it with levels of competence ranging from 'fun' running in the London Marathon to international competition.

It is undoubtedly a serious undertaking, which requires great commitment. There are many benefits from taking part, including the pride of achievement as well as increased self knowledge and understanding of diabetes.

Bibliography

Kibirige M, Court S. Childhood and adolescent diabetes. In: Court S, Lamb WH (eds), *Exercise and Diabetes*. Chichester: John Wiley & Sons, 1997; 273–288.

Ruderman N, Devlin JT (eds). *The Health Professional's Guide to Diabetes and Exercise*. Alexandria, VA: American Diabetes Association, 1995.

Williams C, Devlin JT (eds). *Foods, Nutrition and Sports Performance*. London: E & FN Spon, 1992.

Young JC. Exercise prescription for individuals with metabolic disorders. *Sports Med* 1995; **1**: 43–54.

Useful Addresses

1. American Diabetes Association
   National Service Center
   1660 Duke Street
   Alexandria
   VA 22314, USA

2. British Diabetic Association
   10 Queen Anne Street
   London W1M 0BD, UK
   BDA Careline – Tel: 0171 636 6112

3. The International Diabetic Athletes Association
   1647-B West Bethany Home Road
   Phoenix
   AZ 85015, USA
   E-mail: idaa@diabetes-exercise.org
   www.diabetes-exercise.org

4. The National Sports Institute
   c/o St Bartholomew's Medical College
   Charterhouse Square
   London EC1M 6BQ, UK

10

Diabetes and Specific Sports

Mark Sherlock and **Chris Thompson**

10.1   General Principles

Exercise is an integral part of normal healthy lifestyles. It is increasingly apparent that, while exercise offers a genuine therapeutic intervention in type 2 diabetes, the benefits are less clearly documented for type 1 diabetes. As exercise and participation in active sports become accepted as cornerstone healthy lifestyle choices, there is a need to be aware of specific precautions for the person with diabetes. If exercise occurs without reduction in insulin dose and/or increased carbohydrate intake, hypoglycaemia is very likely. Conversely, exercise in the setting of insulin deficiency is likely to lead to the development of ketoacidosis. The basic principles for making insulin dose reductions, and for taking extra carbohydrate when exercising, were outlined in Chapter 2. When trying to estimate the energy expenditure in different sports, a number of different variables have to be taken into account:

- the type of activity;

- the duration and intensity of exercise;

- the physique of an individual – the greater the body weight, the greater the energy expenditure during exercise;

- the experience of an individual – beginners in many sports, for instance skiing, expend much more energy than those who are experienced;

Exercise and Sport in Diabetes, 2nd Edition   Edited by Dinesh Nagi
© 2005 John Wiley & Sons, Ltd.

- weather conditions – more energy is expended in cold or windy conditions, particularly if the individual is wet and shivering;

- the level of competition – a great deal more effort is likely to be put into a cup final than a training match.

To compare the intensity of different sporting activities, a rating system has been devised which compares the intensity of a given activity with the resting metabolic rate. This is taken to be that of an adult sitting quietly, and is defined as 1 MET (which for an average adult is approximately 3.5 ml oxygen kg^{-1} body weight min^{-1}, or 1 kcal kg^{-1} body weight h^{-1}).[1] The MET value for various activities assesses their intensity in relation to the resting value of 1 MET (Table 10.1). For interest, this table also includes the calorie expenditure per minute and hour while performing different tasks.

By combining the information contained in Table 10.1 with the precise details of insulin dose adjustments given in Chapter 2, it should be possible to calculate the

Table 10.1 Comparative energy expenditure for different sporting activities

Activity	METS	Energy expenditure	
		(kcal min^{-1})	(kcal h^{-1})
Walking (3 mph) Cycling (6 mph) Golf (pulling trolley) Tennis, doubles	3.5–4.0	4–5	240–300
Golf (carrying clubs) Volleyball Walking (4 mph) Mowing lawn, hand mower Roller skating	4.0–6.0	5–6	300–360
Cycling (12 mph) Jogging (5 mph) Tennis, singles Skiing (downhill, vigorous) Aerobics (high impact)	7.0–8.0	7–8	420–480
Cycling, racing Running (6–7 mph) Swimming (crawl, fast) Soccer Rugby Squash	9.0–11.0	10–12	600–660
Rock climbing Canoeing, vigorous Skindiving Running (8–9 mph)	12.0–14.0	12 or more	720 or more

Adapted from Ainsworth et al.,[1] by permission.

alterations of diet and insulin required for most sporting activities. More detailed advice for selected activities now follows.

10.2 Canoeing

Canoeing or kayaking exert considerable demands on carbohydrate stores. Long-distance paddling, particularly on the open sea, can exhaust not only available glucose, but also muscle and hepatic carbohydrate stores, particularly in choppy conditions. This can lead to severe hypoglycaemia, which is likely to repeat unless carbohydrate intake is constantly maintained. In contrast, the short-lived intensity of white-water canoeing can cause rapid falls in blood glucose concentrations. Data from the Firbush Outward Bound diabetes camp indicates that canoeing ranks second only to hillwalking in propensity to cause severe hypoglycaemia. The likelihood of hypoglycaemia is increased if shivering develops secondary to the cold and wet.

As with all sports, it is important to reduce insulin and take extra carbohydrate before starting canoeing. Whilst canoeing, the best way to store carbohydrate for regular 'top-ups' is either to secrete dextrose tablets up the sleeve of a wetsuit or to store chocolate bars in a waterproof bag in the zip pocket of a waterproof overjacket. Because canoeing is particularly prone to causing hypoglycaemia, and because hypoglycaemia can suddenly lead to capsizing the canoe, it is advisable to canoe with a 'buddy' who can recognize and deal with hypoglycaemia and who is proficient in emergency rescue techniques.

Some canoeists suggest that hypoglycaemia is more frequent if insulin is injected into the arms on the morning of the paddle, although the practical importance of this is open to debate (see Chapter 2). Delayed hypoglycaemia on the evening after a paddle is a frequent problem, particularly if paddling has been prolonged, and adequate carbohydrate should be ingested with the evening meal and before bed.

10.3 Golf

Even players themselves often consider golf to be a sport which is not associated with much energy expenditure. Of the sports which we will discuss, it is most likely to be enjoyed by people with type 2 diabetes, who fit the age profile which most commonly plays golf. People with type 2 diabetes who have played golf will, however, be able to confirm that, without precautions, hypoglycaemia is frequent. Although golf does not involve intense effort, the moderate effort is sustained continuously for 4 h or more, and extra energy expenditure occurs when carrying one's own clubs or when playing on a hilly course. In addition, as it is not customary to consume food during a round of golf, the likelihood of developing hypoglycaemia is significant. In fact, players with type 2 diabetes usually find that they need to take additional carbohydrate after the first nine holes. Our recommendation to players with type 2 diabetes is to take substantial carbohydrate prior to a round – a sandwich in the clubhouse, for example – and to top up with readily available carbohydrate, such as sports drinks or bananas, during the round. As many players find that the effects of hypoglycaemia can last for several holes, with loss of concentration, poor swing and erroneous course management decisions, we recommend prophylactic carbohydrate taken two holes before the usual onset of symptoms.

Players who have insulin-treated diabetes should follow the guidelines for low-to-moderate-intensity exercise outlined in Chapter 2, with suitable adjustments on the basis of playing speed, nature of the course (hilly or not), weather conditions (wind, temperature), and whether or not carrying clubs. Table 10.1 may help in assessing the intensity of exertion, but for a 4 h round it may be necessary to reduce pre-prandial insulin by 20–30 per cent, and basal insulin by up to 40–50 per cent, as well as taking extra carbohydrate after nine holes (see Chapter 2).

10.4   Hillwalking

Hillwalking presents a considerable challenge to the individual with type 1 diabetes. The nature of the exercise, which is both prolonged and strenuous, requires not only a reasonable level of physical fitness but also considerable reduction in insulin dose and marked increases in carbohydrate intake to avoid hypoglycaemia. Hillwalking is more likely to cause hypoglycaemia than any other form of outdoor pursuit, and is particularly likely to cause delayed hypoglycaemia in the evening or the night after a hillclimb has been completed. In addition, hillwalking carries the risk of foot blisters, which necessitates appropriate footwear and good foot care.

The following are guidelines for people with insulin-treated diabetes who wish to participate in hillwalking. They are derived from our own experience in leading hillwalking expeditions in Ireland, the Canadian Rockies and Peru, and they should be regarded as additional to general advice about walking and climbing in mountainous country.

1. Good equipment is essential. Appropriate walking boots which fit comfortably minimize the risk of ankle injuries and blistering. In our experience, blisters are best avoided when a pair of thin socks is worn underneath the thick walking socks traditionally worn on the hills.

2. Warm, waterproof over-clothes should be carried, even in good weather, as conditions can change rapidly on the hills. The combination of exercise and

cold-induced shivering quickly lowers blood glucose into the hypoglycaemic range, and it is important not to become cold.

3. It is not recommended that people with diabetes attempt significant climbs alone, and they ideally should climb or walk with someone who is experienced in the recognition and treatment of hypoglycaemia. A note of the intended route and estimated time of return should be left with someone reliable before departure.

4. The reduction in insulin dose required to avoid hypoglycaemia varies widely between individuals and depends to some extent on the preceding glycaemic control; patients who are not well controlled may develop marked hyperglycaemia and ketosis if insulin dosages are reduced by too much. Advice must be given on an individual basis, but the experience of the Firbush Project (Chapter 7) shows that insulin dose needs to be reduced by 25–30 per cent on average. This applies equally to the dose of insulin on the evening after completing a climb, in order to avoid delayed hypoglycaemia, particularly nocturnal hypoglycaemia. Nocturnal hypoglycaemia, occurring without warning, is more likely to occur if there have been hypoglycaemic attacks during the day. Insulin analogues, which can be injected immediately before eating without detriment to post-prandial blood glucose control, are proving very useful in control of blood glucose concentrations during hillwalking. Climbers on conventional soluble insulin face the dilemma of injecting as recommended, half an hour before eating, and risking hypoglycaemia while walking or climbing to the meal site, or injecting just before eating, in conflict with medical advice. In practice, most climbers opt for safety with the latter option, but the availability of insulin analogues eradicates this dilemma and many patients with insulin-treated diabetes who are regular walkers or climbers have elected to switch to insulin analogues (see Chapter 8). Some people with diabetes have recently altered their precautions when adjusting for hillwalking to adopt an 'exercise on insulin' approach. This entails a smaller reduction in insulin dose, of 15–20 per cent, but a marked increase in intake of easily absorbed carbohydrate, to maintain blood glucose concentrations in the safe range. Experienced walkers feel the higher insulin levels protect against exercise-induced ketosis and improve glucose uptake during exercise, improving performance. There is no published data comparing performance in this situation, and we recommend it only for experienced walkers used to regular monitoring and adjustment.

5. Hillwalking requires considerable energy expenditure, and carbohydrate intake should be increased to provide the necessary fuel and to avoid hypoglycaemia. It is crucially important to have a high-carbohydrate breakfast. The traditional eggs, bacon and sausage breakfast does not provide sufficient carbohydrate, and

breakfast should include cereal and toast, with baked beans or porridge to give a warm start in cold weather. Calorific intake needs to be maintained while walking and we find that a mixture of bananas, raisins, energy bars and chocolate provides a palatable and easily portable variety. Formal meals, such as lunch, should be bigger than usual, and it is important to stress the need for a decent evening meal and a snack before bed to prevent nocturnal hypoglycaemia. Fluid – water is preferable, although isotonic drinks are popular – should also be carried in quantities adequate for the duration of the climb and prevailing climate.

6. Blood glucose monitoring is an integral part of playing sport for people with diabetes, but it is essential that blood glucose should be checked regularly during hillwalking, in view of the high risk of hypoglycaemia. Blood glucose should always be checked before ascending a hill and urinary ketones measured if the blood glucose is greater than $17\,\text{mmol}\,l^{-1}$. Hill climbing should not be attempted while insulin-deficient, as ketones are rapidly generated leading to muscle cramps, polyuria and exhaustion. If small amounts of ketones are present a small bolus of soluble insulin should be taken, but if anything more than trace ketonuria is detected, consideration should be given to abandoning the climb.

10.5   Extreme Altitude Mountaineering

Extreme altitude mountaineering is defined as an ascent in excess of 5000 m. With the explosion in charity expeditions to exotic locations and the ease of access to remote mountain ranges, it is increasingly common for diabetes care providers to be asked for advice by people with diabetes attempting extreme altitude mountaineering. In people with diabetes, extreme altitude mountaineering presents a number of physiological and technical challenges. Acute mountain sickness (AMS) is very common at extreme altitude, and is associated with headache, anorexia, fatigue, ataxia, sleep disturbance and retinal haemorrhages. AMS occurs in more than 50 per cent of people at a height of 4559 m or more. Much of the advice which we offer to diabetic climbers is based on data which we collected on the Diabetes Federation of Ireland Expedition to Kilimanjaro.[2,3]

Specific advice

Like hillwalking, extreme altitude mountaineering requires a higher carbohydrate intake, lower insulin dose and increased fluid intake. In a cohort of 16 patients with type 1 diabetes who climbed Mount Kilimanjaro, the average reduction in insulin dose was 49.3 per cent.[2,3] However, the proportion of blood glucose concentrations between the target 6–14 mmol l^{-1} was only 50 per cent, which emphasizes the difficulty in maintaining euglycaemia during sustained exercise at extreme altitude. The highest risk of hypoglycaemia was in the first 2 days of the expedition as, after this, insulin doses were decreased accordingly. In addition, as the anorexia associated with AMS renders adequate carbohydrate intake difficult, hypoglycaemia may also occur at higher altitudes later during a prolonged ascent. During the Kilimanjaro expedition one individual substantially reduced insulin dosage to compensate for poor food intake secondary to anorexia, and developed ketoacidosis, which required evacuation from the mountain. Therefore it is suggested that people with diabetes should have a pre-expedition training schedule which allows familiarization with insulin dose adjustment and carbohydrate and fluid intake during sustained exercise.

In patients using short acting insulin analogues, the administration of insulin is better delayed until the end of the meal as at altitude there seems to be a delay in carbohydrate absorption and a more rapid onset of insulin action.

The data from the Kilimanjaro expedition indicated that there was no inherent increase in the risk of AMS, as measured by the well-validated Lake Louise scoring system,[4] in people with diabetes. However, some of the symptoms of AMS, such as headache and light-headedness, mimic the symptoms of hypoglycaemia. In addition, the difficulty in maintaining carbohydrate intake when anorexia occurs is more problematic for people with diabetes.

Acetazolamide (carbonic anhydrase inhibitor) is used frequently in the prevention of AMS. One patient who developed ketoacidosis on the Kilimanjaro expedition had prolonged acidosis after clearance of urinary ketones. The patient had been taking acetazolamide for prevention of AMS and it is possible that the acetazolamide worsened acidosis in this case. In the literature there are two separate reports of groups of people with diabetes climbing higher than 5000 m, one climbing Mount Kilimanjaro (5895 m)[2,3] and the other the Aconcagua (6950 m).[5] In the Aconcagua ascent, acetazolamide was not administered, although the acclimatization period was longer than that of the Kilimanjaro group, who did use acetazolamide. Therefore, a longer acclimatization period during ascent may obviate the need for acetazolamide.

At extreme altitude and extremes of temperature, the performance of blood glucose meters can be variable. In the Kilimanjaro study the trend was toward low readings and at a height of 4500 m the measured readings were 60–80 per cent of standard solution concentrations.[2,3] At a height of 5900 m, one-third of the participants' meters did not give readouts. Other studies have confirmed the unreliable performance of blood glucose meters at altitude.[6–8] It is estimated that, with each 330 m elevation, there is a 2 per cent underestimation in glucose.[9] Therefore, elevated blood glucose levels at high altitudes and low temperatures are an underestimation. However in the Aconcagua (6950 m) expedition this problem seemed to be overcome by carrying devices in bags under garments and next to the skin, in order to minimize the exposure to low temperatures.

The risk of retinal haemorrhage is high at extreme altitude, due to retinal vessel hypoxia. At heights in excess of 5000 m one-third of climbers develop retinal haemorrhages. Two out of 16 of the diabetic climbers on the Kilimanjaro expedition (and three out of 22 non-diabetic climbers) developed new retinal haemorrhages.[2,3] People with diabetic retinopathy which is more severe than background, should be informed that the risk of worsening retinopathy is significant at extreme altitude.

People with diabetes must take a decision about participating in extreme altitude mountaineering on the basis of sound caution concerning potential risks. Perhaps the key advice is that the risk of ketoacidosis is closely linked to the development of AMS. Measures to reduce the risk of AMS are therefore crucial – and the most important is gradual ascent.

10.6   Rowing

Competition rowing is among the most strenuous activities listed in Table 10.1. The precautions required for rowers with diabetes are generally similar to the advice given for canoeing. Rowing is generally an 'explosive' effort, usually sustained for about 6 min and not maintained for longer than 20–30 min at full intensity. While it is somewhat less likely than canoeing to involve complete immersion, there is still a requirement to have a safe, dry, accessible stowage place for glucose tablets or drinks for use in an emergency.

For competitions, the main need is to ensure that diabetes is under reasonable control (blood glucose <14 mmol 1^{-1} and no ketones), and that a high-carbohydrate meal is taken about 2 h before the event, with a moderate reduction of short-acting insulin before the race. Training sessions are likely to be of longer duration, and may require greater reductions in insulin dose both before and after the session.

Case history: Steve Redgrave

Olympic oarsman Steve Redgrave was holder of the gold medal for coxless pairs (won at Atlanta, 1996), when he suddenly developed diabetes in October 1997, at the age of 36.[2] Although the onset was quite dramatic, and blood glucose was in excess of 20 mmol 1^{-1}, he had a family history of type 2 diabetes, and eventually turned out to have developed this type himself. The condition could be controlled by sulfonylurea treatment, but this produces a constant stimulus to insulin secretion, which did not suit the variable demand for insulin imposed by Steve's training regime. He prefers to control his diabetes with five or six daily injections of the short-acting insulin analogue lispro (Humalog, see Chapter 8), because the typical twice-daily injection routine used for people with type 2 diabetes was also too inflexible. Steve initially considered abandoning his plans to continue competing until the Olympics in 2000, but eventually decided that he was not going to let diabetes make this decision for him.

He finds that Humalog gives him flexibility together with precise control of blood glucose. 'Ideally, I eat what I want, the insulin acts and is out of my system before the next training session. But when you are training all day, it can be hard to find a time to inject that won't affect the next training session, so I tend to balance it with the last injection of the day, snacking before bed. The first session's the hardest, so if I have got the glucose level right overnight, I don't need any insulin in the morning, because the training brings the levels down anyway. Before the second session I have a snack and do a test; as it tends to be less physical, and glucose levels fall less, I take a little insulin.'

He carries glucose tablets or drinks on the water, but has not had problems while training. 'Long distance races will be the biggest challenge, and on those days I reckon I will have to allow a higher blood glucose level.' Knowledge that other people have overcome the problems associated with diabetes and elite sport has been helpful. 'There's a guy with diabetes in the German Eight who came fourth at the last world championships, which helped to prove that you can still compete at high levels.'

As an athlete, Steve was already aware of his dietary needs, and found diabetes perhaps less of an imposition than other people. 'It's definitely an advantage being a sportsman. You have to be very disciplined about your whole lifestyle. Diabetes is just another part of the equation. It's not difficult – it's a pain in the neck, but that's all really.'

10.7 Soccer and Rugby

Soccer and rugby rarely present problems to people with insulin-treated diabetes. If insulin is reduced – usually by 25–30 per cent – before the game, and extra carbohydrate is taken before playing, at half-time, and at the end of the game, hypoglycaemia is not common. Most players take carbohydrate, usually in the form of dextrose tablets or isotonic drinks, to be left on the touchline in case of hypoglycaemia during a game. Delayed hypoglycaemia tends to be more of a problem, particularly after hard, prolonged evening training sessions; training is often more intense than the match itself, where there may be periods of rest. As evening training often terminates with alcoholic beverages, the combination of hard exercise, alcohol and delayed or missed meals can lead to significant nocturnal hypoglycaemia. Hypoglycaemia can be avoided by ensuring that a meal rich in complex carbohydrate – preferably pasta-based – is taken after training has finished and by moderating alcohol intake. There are a number of key role models in professional soccer who have played to international level despite the perceived handicap of diabetes, including Danny McGrain (Celtic and Scotland) and Alan Kernaghan (Middlesborough and Ireland).

10.8 Tennis

Although tennis is characterized by periods of high-intensity exercise, the metabolic demands of even high-level competition are those of moderate-intensity, sustained exercise.[10] Table 10.1 highlights the difference between singles and doubles, the former having an energy expenditure equivalent to 8 METS, and the latter being equivalent to 6 METS. Tennis rarely causes major metabolic disturbances in people with insulin-treated diabetes, although, as with other sports, due consideration has to be given to variables such as time in relation to last meal and insulin injection, type and dosage of insulin, amount and type of food taken, duration and intensity of match, and time of day.

Hypoglycaemia occurring during, or up to 4–6 h after, the match is the most common problem, and is relatively easily avoided by a pre-match check of blood glucose and by taking readily absorbed carbohydrate before, during and after the match. It is also advisable to make modest reductions in the dose of insulin, especially for prolonged matches, following the principles outlined in Chapter 2.

10.9 Sub-Aqua (Scuba) Diving

People with insulin-treated diabetes were at one time prevented from underwater swimming. However, a study which examined the effect of diving to depths of 27 m, simulated in a hyperbaric chamber, showed that there was no increase in risk of hypoglycaemia in patients with well-controlled type 1 diabetes (defined as no grade 4 hypoglycaemic events within the last 12 months, a HbA1c <9% and no complications of type 1 diabetes). The authors concluded that it should be safe to allow people with well-controlled type 1 diabetes to undertake scuba diving.[11] The regulations of the British Sub-Aqua Club have now been changed to allow people with insulin-treated diabetes to dive, provided certain criteria are fulfilled. A medical referee must certify that the diver with diabetes is fit and in good health. Their diving buddy should be someone who is either a regular diving partner who is familiar with diabetes, or a trained medic or paramedic. In addition, if diving in cold water a wet suit ≥5 mm thickness should be worn in order to reduce shivering and the propensity to hypoglycaemia.

Following a survey of 18 experienced divers with type 1 diabetes, the following safety tips have been recommended:[12]

1. more frequent blood glucose monitoring on day of dive;

2. increased carbohydrate intake on day of dive and food intake 1 h pre-dive;

3. avoidance of alcohol for 24 h pre-dive;

4. liquid form of glucose carried on dive, e.g. Hypostop gel;

5. people with diabetes should dive with a regular dive buddy who is fully aware of the signs and management of a hypoglycaemic episode;

6. blood glucose pre-dive should be >8 mmol l^{-1};

7. if blood glucose is <8 mmol l^{-1} then short-acting carbohydrate should be ingested pre-dive.

10.10 Skiing

Skiing is associated with increased carbohydrate requirements due to both physical activity and hypothermia. The importance of appropriate equipment and clothing cannot be overemphasized. In one study, which reported the experience of a cohort of 43 young people with diabetes while skiing, there were no serious hypoglycaemic episodes. On average the insulin dose reduction was 20 per cent, with increased dose reductions for people who had an advanced skiing ability, were previously very inactive or who frequently had hypoglycaemias. The effects of excess alcohol, which are an integral part of many skiing holidays, were offset by reduction of insulin dosage and an increase in evening carbohydrate intake.[13]

10.11 Restrictions Imposed by Sports Governing Bodies

In general, our philosophy is to encourage participation in all forms of sport and exercise, but it should be acknowledged that there are restrictions placed by sports governing bodies on participation by people treated with insulin. The following section summarizes current recommendations and includes some useful websites from which further information can be obtained.

No restrictions

The following sports have no restrictions imposed by sports governing bodies: angling, archery, badminton, baseball, basketball, billiards, bowls, camogie, caving (provided group leader is informed), cricket, croquet, cycling, fencing, football, Gaelic football, gymnastics, handball, hockey (need to notify coach), horse riding, hurling, judo, modern pentathlon, mountaineering, polo, rounders, rowing, rugby league, rugby union (inform team doctor), sailing, shooting, skiing, squash, surfing, swimming, tchouk-ball, table tennis, tennis, weightlifting, wind-surfing and wrestling.

Participation banned

There are a small number of sports in which people with diabetes are not allowed to participate, and these are summarized in Table 10.2.

Table 10.2   Restrictions imposed by sports governing bodies on participation for people with insulin-treated diabetes

Some restrictions	Total ban on participation
Ballooning	Bobsleigh
Gliding	Boxing
Motorcycle racing	Flying
Parachuting	Horse racing
Power boat racing	Motor racing
Rowing	Paragliding
Underwater swimming	

Boxing

The Amateur Boxing Association does not allow people with diabetes, whether on insulin, oral hypoglycaemic agents or diet alone, to box. All applicants must have a medical before boxing and if diabetes is diagnosed the applicant is automatically disqualified. The obvious concern is the ability of an individual to mount a defence if they become hypoglycaemic; this does not, however, prevent people with diabetes participating in other contact sports such as judo and karate. However, as the sport is separated into weight divisions, there is a serious concern over the effects that 'wasting' (losing weight before a bout in order to fight in a certain weight bracket) would have on control of diabetes. The Amateur Boxing Association does run a beginners' achievement course that involves no physical contact, but is designed to promote exercise and develop moral and ethical behaviour, and this is open to people with diabetes (www.britishboxing.net and www.bbbofc.com).

Flying

People with insulin-treated diabetes will not be issued with a flying licence, although people on oral hypoglycaemics can hold a private licence but must fly with a co-pilot (www.pfa.org.uk and www.caa.co.uk).

Parachuting

Parachute jumping is restricted to tandem jumping, although if an individual develops diabetes after he/she has already been jumping, the case will be judged by the British Parachute Association on individual merit (www.Bpa.org.uk).

Motor racing

Insulin-treated diabetics are banned from holding a competitive driving licence and so they cannot compete in motor racing (www.msauk.org).

Bobsleigh

It is unlikely that insulin-treated diabetics would be passed as bobsleigh drivers in the medical examinations that all potential competitors must have (www.british-bobsleigh.com).

Participation restricted

A number of sporting bodies impose certain restrictions upon people with diabetes; some of these are simply to satisfy insurance requirements, whereas some are designed to ascertain individual suitability to participate. The sports of sub-aqua diving and horse racing are good examples of how attitudes to people with diabetes are changing, and how the regulations imposed by sports governing bodies can be changed by the pressure of well-balanced arguments and sound medical advice.

Athletics

There are no restrictions presuming the person with a diabetes has consulted with a doctor prior to participation in a specific sport. It is of note that insulin is now a banned substance due to its abuse as a performance enhancer and therefore all people with diabetes need to provide a letter from their doctor stating they need to use insulin to treat their diabetes (www.ukathletics.org.uk).

Judo

There are no restrictions imposed by the British Judo Association upon people with diabetes. Application forms are used by all martial arts clubs and, if applicants declare that they have a 'chronic condition' such as diabetes, a medical certificate, mainly for insurance purposes, is required from a qualified medical practitioner which clears the applicant to participate (www.britishjudo.org.uk).

Sub-aqua diving

People with insulin-treated diabetes were at one time prevented from underwater swimming, but the regulations of the British Sub-Aqua Club were changed so that people with insulin-treated diabetes could dive, provided certain criteria could be fulfilled (www.bsac.com, www.saa.org.uk and www.scotsac.com).

The UKSDMC have a number of criteria which need to be satisfied before people with diabetes can dive:

- there should have been no serious hypoglycaemic episode in the last year;

- the patient should not have been hospitalized for reasons related to diabetes in the last year;

- the person's diabetologist must feel that diabetes control is satisfactory;

- the doctor must be able to state that the diver is mentally and physically fit to dive;

- there should be no long-term complications such as neuropathy, nephropathy, cardiovascular disease and retinopathy beyond background retinopathy.

Horse racing

People on insulin are not permitted to become jockeys, but each case is examined individually (www.thejockeyclub.co.uk).

Ballooning

The British Balloon and Airship Club require a declaration of fitness to be completed and countersigned by the individual's own doctor, who is therefore completely empowered to decide on the fitness of an individual (ww.bbac.org).

Canoeing

Although there are no restrictions on a person with diabetes canoeing, an individual with diabetes can be granted a coaching award only if they undergo an annual medical review. A general practitioner or consultant must confirm that their diabetes is stable and undertakes to notify the British Canoe Union of any change in circumstance. If an existing coaching scheme member develops diabetes, they will be temporarily suspended pending stabilization of diabetes (www.bcu.org.uk).

Gliding

People with diabetes are allowed to fly as a glider pilot if a declaration of fitness is endorsed by a general practitioner or an authorized medical examiner, but should not expect to become instructors, enter competition or undertake long cross-country flights (www.glidimg.co.uk).

Motorcycling

Motorcycling is relatively open to people with diabetes. Participation in special events requires a medical certificate to be produced; the certificate asks if the participant has diabetes, but if the diabetes is stable and the subject is not subject to frequent hypos, they should be passed as fit to race. Medicals are required every 5 years. No medicals are required for trials, endurance, drag and sprint competitions, except at international level (www.acu.org.uk).

Rowing

Surprisingly, although there are no restrictions on membership of the Great Britain Rowing Team, the Amateur Rowing Association require insulin-treated diabetics to be under regular medical supervision; participation is allowed if glycaemic control is good and the subject is 'free of hypoglycaemic attacks' (www.ara-rowing.org).

Powerboats

Individuals interested in power boat racing are assessed on the basis of previous sailing experience, glycaemic control and frequency of hypoglycaemia, but are likely to be passed fit to race if these parameters are deemed appropriate (www.rya.org.uk).

Triathlon

The British Triathlon Association imposes no restrictions upon people with diabetes, but insists that the fact that one has diabetes should be written on the back of the race number and that one of the medical professionals in attendance should be aware that the individual has diabetes (www.britishtriathlon.org).

10.12   Conclusion

The American Diabetes Association 2001 Position statement asserts that 'all levels of exercise, including leisure activities, recreational sports, and competitive professional performance, can be performed by people with type 1 diabetes who do not have complications and are in good glucose control.' The vast majority of sports are entirely open to people with diabetes and impose no restrictions upon participation. However, for each individual, careful consideration must be given to alterations in carbohydrate intake and insulin administration to allow safe participation. Some sports, such as extreme altitude mountaineering, have no restrictions for diabetes but are clearly considerable challenges, with significant risks for even the fittest and most committed athlete with diabetes. If in doubt, national sport-governing bodies should be contacted; Diabetes UK will supply an up-to-date list of addresses of all sports associations together with regulations and restrictions on request.

References

1. Ainsworth BE, Haskell WL, Leon AS *et al*. Compendium of physical activities: classification of energy costs of human physical activities. *Med Sci Sports Exerc* 1993; **25**: 71–80. [Quoted in *Balance* no. 164, 13–15 July/August 1998. London: British Diabetic Association Publications.]
2. Moore K, Vizzard N, Coleman C, McMahon J, Hayes R, Thompson CJ. Extreme altitude mountaineering and type 1 diabetes; the Diabetes Federation of Ireland Kilimanjaro expedition. *Diab Med* 2001; **18**: 749–755.
3. Moore K, Thompson C, Hayes R. Diabetes and extreme altitude mountaineering. *Br J Sports Med* 2001; **35**: 83.
4. Roach RC, Bartsch P, Hackett PH *et al*. The Lake Louise acute mountain sickness scoring system. In *Hypoxia and Molecular Medicine*, 1st edn, Sutton JR, Houston CS, Coates G (eds). Burlington, VT: Queen City Printers, 1993; 52–59.
5. Admetlla J, Leal C, Ricart A. Management of diabetes at high altitude. *Br J Sports Med* 2001; **35**: 282–283.
6. Giordano N, Trash W, Hollenbaugh L *et al*. Performance of seven glucose testing systems at high altitude. *Diabes Educ* 1989; **15**: 444–448.
7. Pecchio O, Maule S, Migliardi M *et al*. Effects of exposure at an altitude of 3000 m on performance of glucose meters. *Diabetes Care* 2000; **23**: 129–131.
8. Gautier JF, Bigard AX, Douche P *et al*. Influence of simulated altitude on the performance of five glucose meters. *Diabetes Care* 1996; **19**: 1430–1433.
9. Fink KS, Christensen DB, Ellsworth A. Effect of high altitude on blood glucose meter performance. *Diabet Technol Ther* 2002; **4**(5): 627–635.

10. Bergeron MF, Maresh CM, Kraemer WJ, Abraham A, Conroy B, Gabaree C. Tennis: physiological profile during match play. *Int J Sports Med* 1991; **12**: 474–479.
11. Edge CJ, Grieve AP, Gibbons N, O'Sullivan F, Bryson P. Control of blood glucose in a group of diabetic scuba divers. *Undersea Hyperb Med* 1997; **24**(3): 201–207.
12. Kruger D, Owen S, Whitehouse F. Scuba diving and diabetes. *Diabetes Care* 1995; **18**(7): 1074.
13. Chadwick J, Brown KGE. A party of 43 young people with diabetes go skiing. *Diab Med* 1992; **9**: 671–673.

11

Becoming and Staying Physically Active

Elizabeth Marsden and Alison Kirk

11.1 Recommendations for Physical Activity and Exercise

The benefits of regular exercise for people with diabetes have been outlined in Chapter 4. During recent years, diabetes health professionals, the World Health Organization, many books, journals and magazines, have promoted the idea that regular exercise should be undertaken by people with diabetes if they are to stay healthy and fit. The traditional exercise prescription for both health gains and physical fitness benefits has been based on guidelines by the American College of Sports Medicine first produced in 1978 and reviewed again in 1990 and in 1998.[1] These guidelines stated that a minimum of at least 3×20 min sessions per week of moderate to vigorous intensity exercise (60–80 per cent of maximum heart rate) should be undertaken.

The word 'exercise' has certain connotations and evokes strongly held views amongst both patients and health professionals.[2] The traditional view has been that, in order to do any good, exercise must be hard, and therefore an activity in which only young people are likely to engage. A large number of men and women have also been deterred by popular images of sport and exercise, as they do not consider themselves to be sporty types.[3] The 'old' view of exercise may be partly to blame for the low participation levels presently seen in diabetic populations. A survey of west of Scotland diabetic clinics was carried out to establish the percentage of regular exercisers among the insulin-dependent population and showed that only 28 per cent regarded themselves as regular exercisers, compared with 41 per cent of NHS staff and 32 per cent of further education college students.[4] Research demonstrates that only 20–30 per cent of people with type 2

Exercise and Sport in Diabetes, 2nd Edition   Edited by Dinesh Nagi
© 2005 John Wiley & Sons, Ltd.

diabetes do enough activity to improve and maintain their health.[5] Although these figures for participation levels are similar to the general population, research suggests that people with diabetes experience a significantly greater frequency of relapse from physical activity programmes.[6] Furthermore, the greatest number of people with diabetes report low adherence to exercise recommendations, compared with other diabetic self-care behaviours.[7]

Early views concerning the health benefits of exercise were focused on obtaining a training effect for fitness. They recommended activity intensity exceeding 60 per cent of maximum heart rate to lower lipids and control diabetes and obesity. These levels of activity are likely to be both inappropriate and unrealistic for a sedentary population and it is no surprise that there is a high drop-out rate and poor compliance. Fortunately, there is now ample evidence that low- to moderate-intensity activities performed regularly and frequently will have long-term health benefits and lower the risk of cardio-vascular disease.[8] In Scotland, the Physical Activity Task Force[9] has recently reported similar findings, and recommended that the greater health gains occur when sedentary people become and stay moderately active. They report that, in the general population of Scotland, 41 people die every week of the year from being inactive. This could be negated if inactive people were to accumulate approximately 30 min of activity most days, such as brisk walking, stair climbing, gardening and household chores. It is therefore necessary to re-examine the information given to sedentary people with diabetes regarding exercise and physical activity. A strategy for encouraging people with diabetes to take up physical activity is more likely to succeed if the message is aimed at goals and activities that are desirable and also obtainable by this population.

11.2   Essential Attributes of a Physical Activity Programme for People with Diabetes

Casperson, et al.[10] attempted to clarify the terms 'physical fitness', 'exercise' and 'physical activity' because they are often misused and confused in both writing and conversation. Physical fitness is defined as a set of attributes (e.g. cardio-respiratory fitness, muscular strength and flexibility) that people have or achieve that relates to the ability to perform physical activity. Physical fitness is mainly determined by physical activity behaviour, although genetic contributions play a variable role.[11] Exercise is planned and structured and tends to involve repetitive movement, done to improve or maintain one or more components of physical fitness. Physical activity, however, is any movement produced by skeletal muscle that results in energy expenditure of 5–7 calories per minute.[9] Good exercise and physical activity programmes share basic ingredients. Although the intensity of an exercise programme in order to enhance fitness is necessarily higher, both should result in health benefits.[8] A balanced programme, containing components of flexibility, aerobic and muscular endurance work is desirable. Programmes may also contain speed and muscular strength work for those involved in specific sports which require training in these components.

Flexibility

Insufficient attention is paid to flexibility as most believe it to be relatively unimportant. Inflexible joints, particularly in older people, can cause a great deal of difficulty in performing ordinary daily tasks, such as getting out of a chair, or even crossing a road before the green man turns red. Good flexibility is the ability to move joints comfortably through their whole range, thus allowing smooth and effective movements in sporting activities and daily tasks. It also helps to prevent injury from muscle pulls. Flexibility, like the other components of a good programme, will be lost during periods of inactivity and should therefore be regularly practised.

Aerobic capacity

The aerobic component of a physical activity programme is important, especially for people with diabetes, as it challenges the cardio-vascular component, and there is now much evidence to show the protective value of aerobic exercise in the cardio-vascular system.[12]

Muscular endurance and muscular strength

Strength training may be designed either to lift the maximum weight in a single effort (muscular strength) or to lift sub-maximal loads for a longer period of time (muscular endurance). Muscular endurance is more important for most sporting activities, to carry out everyday tasks comfortably and even to maintain a pain-free upright position. Research has also demonstrated strength training to be important for improving glucose metabolism in people with diabetes.[13]

A balanced exercise or physical activity programme should contain each of the three most important components – flexibility, aerobic component and muscular endurance.

11.3 Preparation for Exercise

Ready to start?

Before embarking on an activity programme, a sedentary person with diabetes will need support in several ways. Firstly, a basic understanding of how exercise will affect his/her treatment and daily diabetes management is essential. This will require professional advice which is unlikely to be achieved in the context of a busy routine diabetes clinic. It will need a specific appointment with the person responsible for giving exercise advice in the clinic. The advice given should include a brief summary of the known benefits, risks and type of physical activity suitable for this individual. Insulin-treated patients will need detailed instructions for monitoring blood sugar and adjusting food and insulin in relation to exercise (see Chapter 2). The professional giving this advice should have a detailed knowledge of associated conditions, such as heart disease and specific complications of diabetes, which are relevant to increasing physical activity. Formal exercise testing, that is on a treadmill, as a preliminary check before entering an exercise–activity programme, is rarely thought to be necessary in UK clinics, and any risks are considered to be slight as long as there is a gradual build up of physical activity, with instructions to report any problems.

Best foot forward . . .

Once the would-be exerciser has been given medical approval, and has a sound understanding of the effects of physical exercise, he or she will require a degree of patience in starting slowly and comfortably. Physical activity can be of value only if it becomes a regular part of someone's life. Aiming too high at the start is likely to result in discomfort, injury or ill health, and therefore disappointment, frustration and poor compliance. To avoid these early setbacks, a low-intensity activity at the outset, with gradual build-up of activity, is strongly recommended.

The next stage of preparation for exercise–activity is to consider the usual lifestyle and to estimate whether it will be easier to accommodate small bouts of physical activity, which will add up to 30–60 min a day, or whether specific exercise sessions, several times a week, are easier to fit into what is probably already a busy schedule. Whatever decision is made, each session should include flexibility, aerobic activity and muscular endurance. It is also important to decide whether the aim of an exercise programme is to gain fitness and health benefits, or health benefits alone. If both fitness and health benefits are required, then a target heart rate of between 65 and 85 per cent maximum for about 20 min per session and at least three times a week should be the aim. Taking the pulse rate about half way through the exercise session is important (this is described in more detail later in this chapter). As a guide to the intensity level of the exercise, it is also helpful to ask oneself whether the exercise feels hard or easy.[14] In order to gain fitness, the exercise should feel 'hard'. It may be helpful to have a baseline fitness test at a gym or human performance laboratory. The instructor will be able to advise at what level to start and when to return for a follow-up test, which will show whether the exercise programme is working for increased fitness. It is currently not known what level of activity is required for health benefits alone, as the dose–response equation is complex: 'Dose response relationships with physical activity are poorly described for many health outcomes. The need for more research on this topic is clear' (Hardman and Stensel,[12] p. 247).

However, since it is recognized that keeping sedentary people active is extremely important for their health, working at a comfortable level of intensity is the best rule of thumb, that is, up to 60 per cent maximum heart rate and a feeling that the exercise is 'somewhat hard', but certainly not 'hard'. For some people with diabetes, even moderate intensity activity will be impossible, and the basic rule must be that any increase in physical activity is desirable and goals need to be set accordingly.

... And off we go!

Warm-up

Any period of activity should ideally begin with a warm-up. The importance of warming up is based on sound physiological principles. During the warm-up the temperature of the large muscle groups is increased, which allows increased force and velocity of muscular contraction as well as increased blood and oxygen supply to the fibres. Chemical reactions within the muscle tissue are increased and energy from muscle contraction is increased. Finally the warm-up helps prevent tears and damage to connective tissue and thereby prevents joint injury. Warm-up for a beginner should be at least 10 min and should consist of extremely light large-muscle group activity, such as walking, swinging the arms, easy jogging and gentle movements.

If warm-up is too short or omitted within the first few minutes of starting the main exercise session, the exerciser will feel discomfort, rapid heart rate, heavy breathing and muscular fatigue due to the body's inability to use its aerobic system and its dependence on the anaerobic system.

Flexibility exercises

Once warm-up is completed, the beginner exerciser is advised to engage in some flexibility practice of the large muscle groups. Modern stretching techniques are designed to produce slow and gradual lengthening of the muscles, with the full stretch being held for 15–30 s. Muscles stretched in this way are also relaxed. There are many different kinds of stretching exercises. Appendix 1 illustrates a selection of sequential stretches, beginning with the large group of leg muscles, moving onto muscles of the trunk and finally stretches of the arms and shoulders. For the less mobile and for diabetics with more complications, alternative stretches are illustrated.

Aerobic exercise

Essential aerobic activity is rhythmic, repetitive and causes the muscles to work at a level where they require oxygen for the release of energy. There is a wide selection of activities suitable for the aerobic component of an exercise or physical activity programme. It is best to select those which are appropriate to the individual's needs and which are enjoyable. If, for example, the beginning exerciser is overweight, she or he may feel very uncomfortable performing high impact or jarring activities, such as jogging or work with a skipping rope. He or she may also feel ill-at-ease in a class situation where skimpy and tight clothing is the norm. However, the same individual may feel relaxed and comfortable using a bicycle or rowing machine or walking briskly. A regular exerciser may choose a mixture of swimming, playing football, canoeing or running sports for his programme. Examples of aerobic exercises include brisk walking, cycling, cross country skiing, hillwalking, canoeing, rowing, jogging, swimming and any running game. As muscles, including the heart muscle, become conditioned to activity, it is possible and desirable to work for longer or to increase the intensity over a period of weeks or months.

The intensity of exercise for a training effect can be calculated from the heart rate: '220 – the age' will give an estimate of maximum heart rate in beats per minute. In order for fitness to be improved, the pulse rate should between 65 and 85 per cent maximum heart rate. It is wise to calculate what the heart rate should be for a 10 or 15 s count, as this is easy to take during the exercise session. For example, a 45-year-old woman, who enjoys cycling, has decided to enter a cycle marathon. She would like to target her training programme towards becoming fitter. Using the calculation to find her estimated maximum heart rate ($220 - 45 = 175$ beats per minute), she can work out that, in order to be training hard enough, she will need to cycle so that her heart rate is raised to between 65 and 85 per cent of 175; that is between 114 and 149 beats per minute. If gaining fitness is not as important as gaining health benefits, then the target heart rate may be only between 50 and 60 per cent of the maximum heart rate.

Muscular endurance

Muscular endurance activities also play an important part in the complete exercise or physical activity programme. Without a degree of muscular endurance, simple tasks such as gardening, housework or changing a car tyre can become difficult and may result in injury or muscle strain. There are several training principles that should be understood before embarking on the muscular endurance part of the training programme.

In order to improve muscular endurance, the principle of progressive overload must be applied. The beginning exerciser will be unfamiliar with the load values which he/she is capable of lifting. So it is best to start with fairly light weights. The number of repetitions performed (that is, how many times the same exercise is repeated) is normally around 12 to induce endurance. At the correct load, the individual will find repetitions 10, 11 and 12 hard to complete, but still manageable. At the beginning of an exercise programme, it is best to limit the number of sets of repetitions to one or two to avoid muscle soreness. As the exerciser becomes more able, and muscles become used to endurance, another set of 12 repetitions can be added to the programme. Eventually a full three sets can be performed regularly.

A complete muscle endurance programme will include a wider variety of different types of exercises so that a balance is achieved. Often a person's own body weight serves well as the load in the exercise. Muscular endurance improves in those muscles that are specifically being trained. Most exercisers like to vary their programme for muscular endurance quite frequently and the illustrations given in Appendix 2 offer some examples of those exercises that will result in an all-over body conditioning programme. These have been chosen because no special equipment is required and they can be done anywhere. Exercises can be made progressively more difficult by increasing the level or be increasing the repetitions. It is important to work all of the large muscle groups in any one programme.

Cooling down and post-exercise effects

Once the physical activity session is completed, it is necessary to spend a few minutes cooling down. If the body goes from a state of pumping blood at a much increased rate to stopping suddenly, dizziness, nausea or light-headedness might be experienced. The working muscles push blood back to the heart, but when they stop suddenly, without a period of cooling down, the blood pools in the muscles instead of being forced back to the heart. A transition period is required for transferring from hard muscular work to light muscular work. Cooling down is as important as warming up.

Berg[15] maintained that a good aerobic component leaves the exerciser with diabetes feeling more energetic, vitalized, relaxed and happy after the exercise than before. If varied and enjoyable types of exercise have been chosen, and the sessions have been easily accommodated into the individual's life, then anxiety and stress are lessened – which in turn has a beneficial effect on a person's well-being and quality of life. Self esteem and feelings of achievement add to the feel-good effect. In subjects with diabetes these benefits may also have a positive impact on blood glucose control and the feelings of well-being and self reliance may engage these individuals into taking a more active role in management of the diabetes.

Planning

Choosing how to fit exercise or periods of physical activity into an already busy life does take a great deal of thought and planning. In order to gain either health or fitness benefits, exercise and physical activity must be performed on a regular basis. It may be easier for people with diabetes to achieve a better blood glucose balance when each day's energy expenditure is relatively stable, but the sedentary individual who decides to aim for health benefits by taking short periods of physical activity, such as walking to work or cycling to the shops, adding up to 30 min per day, should remember that a complete programme includes muscular endurance, aerobic and flexibility components. It is likely that the short bursts of physical activity throughout the day will be largely aerobic in nature and provision needs to be made to include some muscular endurance and flexibility components at other times during the week. One of the most difficult problems in exercise and physical activity programmes is to find ways to change behaviour and to 'stay with' physical activity, that is to increase long-term compliance.

11.4   Changing Behaviour

Models of physical activity behaviour change

Sallis and Hovell[16] proposed a framework for studying exercise behaviour. This model, shown in Figure 11.1 identifies that exercise behaviour is not an 'all or none' phenomenon, but rather a dynamic process open to considerable change over time.

A further model which views exercise behaviour as a dynamic process is the transtheoretical model of behaviour change.[17] This model, originally used to explain and predict smoking behaviour, has now been extensively used as a valid and reliable model for assessment of readiness to change physical activity behaviour and as a theoretical framework for physical activity promotion interventions.[18] The model suggests individuals move through stages when changing behaviour. These stages have been labelled pre-contemplation, contemplation, preparation, action and maintenance. A definition of each stage is given in

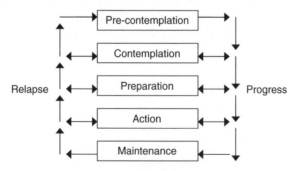

Figure 11.1   The stages of exercise behaviour change[20]

Table 11.1 Stage of exercise behaviour change and appropriate strategies[19,20]

Stage	Definition	Appropriate strategy
Pre-contemplation	Inactive and does not intend to become active in next 6 months	Information/advice on risks of inactivity, benefits of activity
Contemplation	Inactive, but thinking about becoming active in next 6 months	Decision balance (weigh up pros and cons of becoming active) Discuss and overcome barriers
Preparation	Has made some attempts to become more active	Develop realistic activity goals Establish support
Action	Active, but only began in last 6 months	Reinforce successful attempts Re-emphasize experienced benefits, overcome experience barriers
Maintenance	Active for longer than 6 months	Relapse prevention Alternative activities

Table 11.1. As illustrated in Figure 11.1, progression from one stage to another does not always occur in series and individuals can at any time relapse back, or progress forward, one or a number of stages.

Three factors are hypothesized to mediate the process of behaviour change. These are an individual's self efficacy for change (confidence in their ability to change a behaviour), the decisional balance of perceived pros and cons of change and the processes individuals use to modify behaviour.

Using the transtheoretical model of behaviour change

The transtheoretical model proposes that different intervention strategies should be used at different stages of behaviour change to help a person progress to a higher stage or to avoid relapse.[19,20] Table 11.1 outlines a summary of appropriate strategies for each stage of change.

For the person in a pre-contemplation stage of exercise behaviour change, a referral to an exercise class or prescribing an exercise programme is likely to be unsuccessful, and would be a waste of valuable time and resources. At this stage it would be best to present information about the risks of inactivity and the benefits of being more physically active. Providing important information such as the fact that the risk of suffering a cardiovascular event is much higher in an inactive, compared with an active, person with diabetes may be sufficient incentive for a person in the pre-contemplation stage to at least think about becoming more active and thus then progress into a contemplation stage of behaviour change. It will also be helpful if people in a pre-contemplation stage are made aware that, should they wish to become more active in the future, they will have access to adequate support from the exercise counsellor or the person in the diabetes team who is taking responsibility for the promotion of physical activity.

People in either a contemplation or preparation stage of exercise behaviour change are likely to gain most benefit from an intervention such as physical activity counselling (described in detail later). Physical activity counselling should involve the following processes: reviewing current physical activity behaviour, discussing the pros and cons of becoming more active, establishing social support, and developing of realistic physical activity goals. Marsden[2] identified that the barriers to increasing physical activity for people with type 1 diabetes are not diabetes-specific, but are similar to those observed in the general population (i.e. not enough time, other hobbies come first, too lazy, no-one to exercise with). In comparison, research with people with type 2 diabetes has identified that their barriers are diabetes-specific.[21] The most common reported barriers to exercise among people with type 2 diabetes include physical discomfort from exercise, a fear of hypoglycaemia, being too overweight to exercise and lack of support.[21] Perceived benefits of exercise among people with type 1 diabetes are to reduce future diabetic complications, to feel good about oneself and to protect the heart.[2] Perceived benefits among people with type 2 diabetes include improving diabetes control and managing weight.[21]

People with diabetes, like the general population, want to feel good and have fun. In addition, some patients may not realize that there are positive psychological benefits to be gained, such as improving self-confidence and reduced feelings of depression and anxiety. Biddle and Mutrie[22] have suggested that motivations to be physically active may change over a person's lifespan and there is also evidence to suggest different motivating factors between men and women. Young men have been recorded as being more motivated to exercise if they gain social recognition, challenge and competition by doing so; young women, on the other hand, were seeking weight control, enjoyment and physical fitness. Ashford and Biddle[23] surveyed participants at community sports centres to investigate the reasons for undertaking exercise. Older participants were looking for relaxation, social benefits, and health benefits, while challenge and skill-learning motivated younger participants. Other researchers have found important motivating factors to be: improved health;[24] personality of class leader;[25] weight control;[26] better fitness; to socialize and feel better;[27] and medical advice.[28]

For people in either and action or maintenance stage of exercise behaviour, the focus should be on maintaining their current physical activity level and on relapse prevention. It is important that people are aware that relapse is common and that this is not a failure. If relapse does occur, the important issue is to get back to the activity plan as soon as possible. Relapse prevention strategies will involve identifying situations that may have a negative impact on behaviour change, such as a busy work schedule or holidays, and developing ways to prevent relapse during these high-risk situations such as time management or cues to get back to an activity plan after holidays. A review of the person's experienced benefits and barriers to their activity plan will also be useful.

Current application of the transtheoretical model in diabetic populations

The transtheoretical model has been applied successfully to physical activity promotion in the general population. Interventions based on the transtheoretical model, such as stage-matched self-help manuals, motivational interviewing and physical activity counselling are now being increasingly used to promote physical activity. Recent evidence suggests this is also a useful model to promote physical activity behaviour in people with diabetes. Two randomized controlled trials[29,30] have demonstrated a physical activity consultation intervention based on the transtheoretical model to be more effective than standard exercise information for promoting physical activity over the short term (up to 5 weeks) in people with type 1 and type 2 diabetes. More recent research has demonstrated the effectiveness of physical activity counselling based on the transtheoretical model for the longer-term (up to one year) promotion of physical activity in people with type 2 diabetes. In a randomized controlled trial Kirk *et al.*[31–33] found physical activity counselling to be more effective than standard exercise information for promoting and maintaining physical activity over 6 and 12 months in people with type 2 diabetes. Participants randomized to the exercise counselling group also experienced significant improvements in glycaemic control and several cardiovascular risk factors.[31,32]

Including a physical activity advisor within the diabetes team

Promotion of physical activity in current diabetes care is generally inadequate and to date information has mostly been provided in the form of information leaflets or brief advice from the dietician. Whether such advice is provided at all depends on the interests of members of the diabetes team. People with diabetes report receiving the least amount of support, education and encouragement for physical activity compared with any other aspect of diabetes management.[34] Ary *et al.*[7] demonstrated that, although 75 per cent of people with diabetes were told to exercise, only about 20 per cent received written instructions and advice. In comparison 73 per cent were given written instructions and advice about diet. Health professionals are confused about how to promote physical activity to people with type 2 diabetes. Marsden[2] reported that health professionals admit to putting exercise last on the agenda in diabetes management, largely because they do not understand or have knowledge of the possible value that exercise could have for their patients. Perhaps it is not surprising that the majority of people with type 2 diabetes are inactive and attempts to become more active are often met with failure.[5,6]

The Scottish Intercollegiate Guidelines Network (SIGN)[34] on lifestyle management in diabetes recommend that physical activity interventions are individually tailored and diabetes-specific, and to maximize adherence they should provide ongoing support and be tailored to the person's stage of exercise behaviour change. In addition the Health Education Authority[27] actively encourages health care teams to use physical activity counselling. With an increasing number of people being diagnosed with diabetes, in particular type 2 diabetes, and with increasing recognition of physical activity being a fundamental part of diabetes management (see Chapters 4 and 5). The addition of an exercise advisor to current diabetes care is now strongly justified.

Conducting a physical activity consultation

Physical activity consultations take around 30 minutes to conduct and are generally carried out on a one-to-one basis, although they could be adapted to be used with small groups. Physical activity counselling was originally designed to target people in either a contemplation or preparation stage of change, i.e. people who are not meeting current physical activity guidelines but have an intention to become more active.[20] For these individuals the focus of the consultation is to initiate physical activity. This intervention has also been applied effectively to people in other stages of exercise behaviour change, such as people in either an action or maintenance stage. For these individuals a greater emphasis should be placed on maintenance of physical activity and on relapse prevention. Physical activity counselling is a particularly useful intervention for encouraging people with diabetes to become more active. As the intervention is carried out either on an individual basis, or with small groups, physical activity programmes should be tailored to the person's physical and motivational status.

It is important that the health professional chosen to encourage physical activity amongst people with diabetes is a good listener. Whilst one aspect of the health professionals' role is to provide exercise information, advice and encouragement, the skill of hearing what the patient says about his/her own situation, fears, problems, aspirations and goals is of utmost importance.

The general process for conducting a physical activity consultation has been published by Loughlan and Mutrie.[35] Initially it should be established which stage of exercise behaviour change the person fits into. This will determine what strategies should be used within the consultation. Consultations should, however, be individualized to personal needs, therefore the strategies and format used may vary from person to person.

In general, consultations will start by discussing the patient's current physical activity status and establishing the discrepancy between physical activity status and current physical activity recommendations.[118] This can be followed by the completion of a decision balance table. This will involve weighing up the perceived pros and cons of becoming more physically active. This will often involve an explanation of the effectiveness of physical activity in the management of diabetes. This information is of prime importance and should be given in a simple and easily understandable form, beginning with basic principles such as how physical activity will affect their diabetic health and building up to more detailed help such as adjustment of insulin in relation to the type and amount of physical activity to be performed. The overall aim of the decision balance table is to encourage people to perceive more pros than cons for becoming more physically active. Barriers to physical activity should then be discussed. The most frequently cited barriers to physical activity for people with type 1 diabetes are not enough time, other hobbies come first, too lazy and no-one to exercise with.[2] For people with type 2 diabetes they are physical discomfort from exercise, fears of low blood sugar reactions, being too overweight to exercise and lack of support.[21] This section will therefore include a discussion of suitable activities, social support and ways to avoid low blood sugars.

The time barrier can usually be overcome by adding to activities that are already part of the patient's everyday life. It may be useful to make a list of the things the patient does in one day, e.g. walks the dog, catches the bus to work, sits at a desk all day, catches the bus home and watches the TV before walking the dog again. Next suggest how to increase the activity level in each of those areas, e.g. can he/she get off the bus one stop earlier on the way home and walk for a extra 5 min? Can he/she make sure they climb at least one flight of stairs during the lunch break instead of taking the lift to the café? Can he/she walk the dog one block further? By working with the patient's already established lifestyle, extra activity can be added slowly and gradually and does not need to take up a lot of time. Encouraging the patient to substitute inactive tasks with more activity is also beneficial, e.g. wash the car by hand rather than using a car wash.

Not having anyone with whom to exercise with can be very demotivating. Most people find it difficult not to go for that swim when their best friend is standing at the door with towel and goggles all ready to go. Walking to the top of the hill to watch the sunset is far easier if you can chat all the way up with your next door neighbour. Helping your patient to identify an 'exercise buddy' who will agree to work alongside them may be invaluable as a motivational tool. A minority of people, however, prefer to exercise alone.

Goals and rewards are important for adults, as well as children, and for patients in all categories of stage of exercise behaviour change. The next step for the person conducting the physical activity consultation is to find appropriate goals and rewards for the individual. Goals set too high may result in frustration, while goals set too low may result in boredom. Patients in either of these states may relapse and stop being active. It is important to work with the patient when establishing goals. Discuss past and potential new activities and this will identify the person's likes and dislikes in relation to physical activity. Time-phased physical activity goals, including goals for the short-term (1 month), intermediate term (3 months) and long-term (6 months) will help to keep motivation high. Rewards should be linked to the achievement of the goals and may be a prize or treat or something more personal to the patient. Some patients may feel their reward is in performing in the annual show, having taken up tap dancing; others will aim for the London marathon and find their reward is in completing it successfully; yet others will be rewarded when they can manage to walk to the shops and back and still have the energy to make the tea!

The moderate amount of physical activity associated with health benefits (outlined in Chapters 4 and 10) is achievable in most patients with a degree of encouragement and continued support. It is important that people with diabetes are able to identify types of exercise or physical activity that are feasible and enjoyable. The ultimate aim of diabetes care is longevity and quality of life enjoyed by each patient. Physical activity and exercise have an important part to play in realization of these aims.

References

1. ACSM. The recommended quantity and quality of exercise for developing and maintaining cardiorespiratory and muscular fitness, and flexibility in healthy adults. *Med Sci Sports Exerc* 1998; **30**: 975–991.
2. Marsden E. The role of exercise in the wellbeing of people with insulin dependent diabetes mellitus: perceptions of patients and health professionals. Doctoral thesis, Glasgow University, 1996.
3. Biddle S, Mutrie N. *Psychology of Physical Activity*. London: Routledge, 2003.
4. Mutrie N, Loughan C, Campbell M, Marsden E, McCorran T. The transtheoretical model applied to four Scottish populations. *J Sports Sci* 1997; **15**: 100.
5. Hays LM, Clark DO. Correlates of physical activity in a sample of older adults with type 2 diabetes. *Diabetes Care*, **22**: 706–712.
6. Krug LM, Haire-Joshu D, Heady SA. Exercise habits and exercise relapse in persons with non-insulin-dependent diabetes mellitus. *Diabet Educ* 1991; **17**: 185–188.
7. Ary DV, Toobert D, Wilson W, Glasgow RE. Patient perspective on factors contributing to non-adherence to diabetes regimens. *Diabetes Care* 1986; **9**: 168–72.
8. Pate RR, Pratt M, Blair SN, Hashell WL, Macera CA, Bouchard C, Buchner D, Ettinger W, Heath GW, King AC, Kriska A, Lpon AS, Marcus BH, Marris J, Paffenbarger RS, Patrick K, Pollock ML. Rippe JM, Sallis J, Wilmore Jh. Physical activity and public health: a recommendation from the Centers for Disease Control and prevention and the American College of Sports Medicine. *JAMA* 1995; **273**: 402–407.
9. Physical Activity Task Force. *Let's Make Scotland More Active*. London: HMSO, 2003.
10. Casperson CJ, Powell KE, Christenson GM. (1985) Physical activity, exercise and physical fitness: Definitions and distinctions for health related research. *Publ Hlth Rep* 1985; **100**: 126–131.
11. Bouchard C, Perusse L. Physical activity, fitness and health: international proceedings and consensus statement. In *Heredity, Activity Level, Fitness and Health*, Bouchard C, Shepard R, Stephens T (eds). Champaign, IL: Human Kinetics, 1994; 106–118.
12. Hardman A, Stensel D. *Physical Activity and Health*. London: Routledge.

13. Honkola A, Forsen T, Eriksson J. Resistance training improves the metabolic profile in individuals with type 2 diabetes. *Acta Diabetol* 1997; **34**: 245–248.

14. Borg GA. Pshychological bases of perceived exertion. *Med Sci Sport Exerc 1982;* **14**: 377–387.

15. Berg K. *Diabetics' Guide to Health and Fitness*. Champaign IL: Human Kinetics, 1986.

16. Sallis J, Hovell M. Determinants of exercise behaviour. *Exerc Sports Sci Rev* 1990; **18**: 307–330.

17. Prochaska JO, DiClemente CC. Transtheoretical therapy: towards a more integrative model of change. *Psychother Theory Res Pract* 1982; **20**: 161–173.

18. Proshaska JO, Marcus BH. The transtheoretical model: application to exercise. In Advances in Exercise Adherence, Dishman R (ed). Georgia: Human Kinetics, 1994; 161–180.

19. Rollnick S, P Mason, Butler C. *Health Behaviour Change*. London: Churchill Livingstone, 1999.

20. Marcus B, Selby VC, Niaura RS, Rossi JS. The stages of exercise behavior. *Res Q Exerc Sport* 1992; **63**: 60–66.

21. Swift CS, Armstrong JE, Beerman KA, Campbell RK, Pond-Smith D. Attitudes and beliefs about exercise among persons with non-insulin-dependent diabetes. *Diabet Educ* 1995; **21**: 533–540.

22. Biddle S, Mutrie N. Exercise adoption and maintenance. In *Psychology of Physical Activity and Exercise*. London: Springer, 1991; 27–61.

23. Ashford B, Biddle S. Participation in community sports centres: motives and predictors of enjoyment. *J Sports Sci* 1990; 8.

24. Paffenberger RS, Hyde RT, Wing RL. Physical activity and physical fitness as determinants of health and longevity. In Bouchard C, Shephard RJ, Stephens T, Sutton JR, Mcpherson BD (eds). *Exercise Fitness and Health: a Consensus of Current Knowledge*, Champaign, IL: Human Kinetics, 1990; 33–48.

25. Pender NJ, Pender AR. Attitudes, subjective norms and intentions to engage in health research. *Nurs Res* 1986; **35**: 15–18.

26. Rhodes E, Dunwoody D. Physiological and attitudinal changes in those involved in an employee fitness program. *Can J Public Health* 1980; **71**: 331–336.

27. Health Education Authority. *Promoting Physical Activity in Primary Health Care*. London: HEA, 1996.

28. Iverson DC, Fielding JE, Crow RS, Christenson GM. The promotion of physical activity in the United States' population: the status of programmes in medical, worksite, community and school settings. *Publ Hlth Rep* 1985; **100**: 212–1224.

29. Hasler T, Fisher BM, MacIntyre PD, Mutrie N. Exercise consultation and physical activity in patients with type 1 diabetes. *Pract Diab Int* 2000; **17**: 44–48.

30. Kirk AF, Higgins LA, Hughes AR, Fisher M, Mutrie N, Mclean J, MacIntyre P. A randomised controlled trial to study the effect of exercise consultation on the promotion of physical activity in people with type 2 diabetes: a pilot study. *Diab Med* 2001; **18**: 877–883.

31. Kirk A, Mutrie N, MacIntyre P, Fisher M. Effects of a 12-month physical activity counselling intervention on glyceamic control and on the status of cardiovascular risk factors in people with type 2 diabetes. *Diabetologia* 2004; **47**: 821–832.

32. Kirk A, Mutrie N, MacIntyre P, Fisher M. Promoting and maintaining physical activity in people with type 2 diabetes. *Am J Prev Med* 2004; **27**: 289–296.

33. Kirk AF, Mutrie N, MacIntyre P, Fisher M. Increasing physical activity in people with type 2 diabetes. *Diabetes Care* 2003; **26**: 1186–1192.

34. Wilson W, Ary DV, Bigard AX, Glasgow RE, Toobert D, Campbell DR. Psychosocial predictors of self-care behaviors (compliance) and glycemic control in non-insulin-dependent diabetes mellitus. *Diabetes Care* 1986; **9**: 614–622.

35. Loughlan C, Mutrie N. Conducting an exercise consultation: Guidelines for health professionals. *J Inst Health Educ* 1995; **33**: 78–82.

36. Scottish Intercollegiate Guidelines Network. *Management of Diabetes: Lifestyle Management*. SIGN Guideline number 55. Edinburgh: SIGN, 2001.

Appendix 1: Stretching Exercises

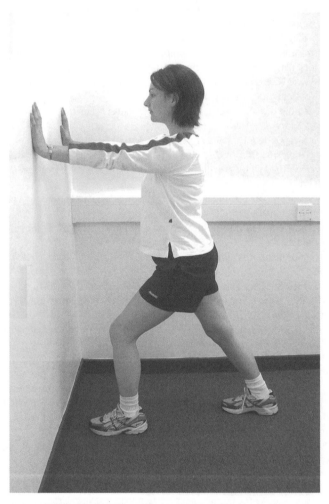

Figure 11.A1   Calf stretch. Face a wall and place both hands at shoulder height on the wall. Both feet are pointing towards the wall. Take the left foot back 2–3 feet, keep the heel flat on the floor. Lean gently forward until the stretch can be felt in the calf muscle. Hold the position for 15–30 s. Slowly change legs and repeat

(a)

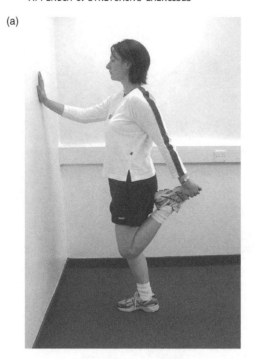

(b)

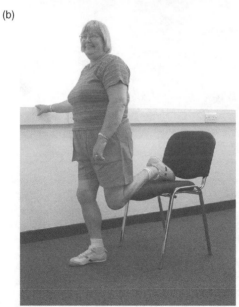

Figure 11.A2 Quadriceps stretch. (a) Stand facing the wall and use one hand to balance. Use the other hand to bring the outside foot backwards towards the bottom. Keep knees fairly close together. To reach a full stretch it may be necessary to push the hips forward. Hold for 15–30 s then stretch the opposite leg. (b) As an easier alternative, instead of holding your foot, support your leg on a chair

(a)

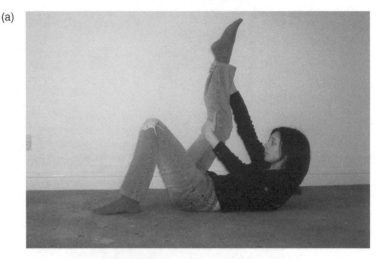

(b)

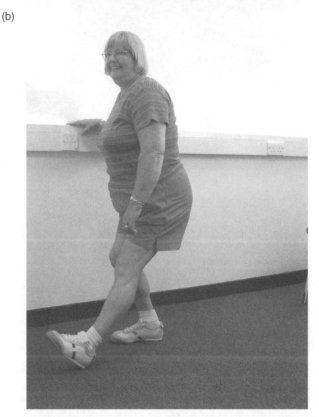

Figure 11.A3   Hamstring stretch. (a) Lying on the floor with the left knee bent, slowly bring the other straightened leg towards the chest. Try to relax the right hamstring as it is being stretched. Hold for 15–30 s. Slowly change legs and repeat. (b) As an easier alternative bring your leg out in front of you and put your heel on the ground. Bend the other leg, lower the hips and push your bottom out behind you. Hold for 15–30 s, then slowly change legs and repeat

(a)

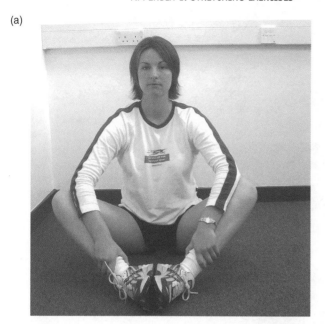

(b)

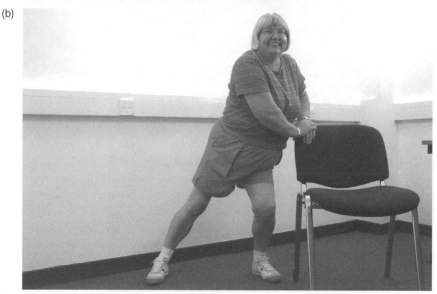

Figure 11.A4 Groin stretch. (a) Sit on the floor with feet apart and backs of the legs on the floor. Slowly walk the fingers forward until a stretch is felt in the groin. Hold for 15–30 s. (b) As an easier alternative stand with your feet wide apart. Keep one leg straight whilst bending the other leg. Move the body over the bent leg. Hold for 15–30 s. To assist with balance this can be done with the support of a chair or wall

(a)

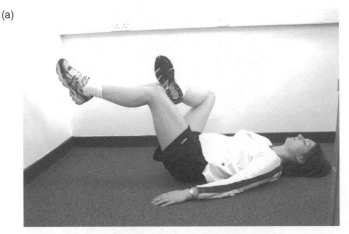

(b)

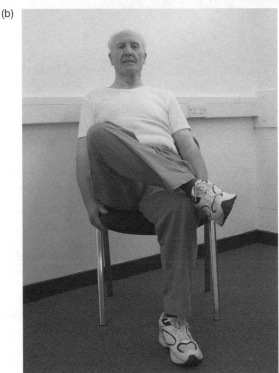

Figure 11.A5   Gluteus maximus stretch. (a) Lying on the floor with the left leg bent, bring the right ankle to rest above the left knee. Slowly lift the left foot from the ground until a stretch can be felt in the right gluteus maximus. Hold for 15–30 s before changing legs. (b) As an easier alternative, sit on a chair and bring the right ankle to rest above the left knee. Slowly lean forward until a stretch can be felt in the right gluteus maximus. Hold for 15–30 s before changing legs

(a)

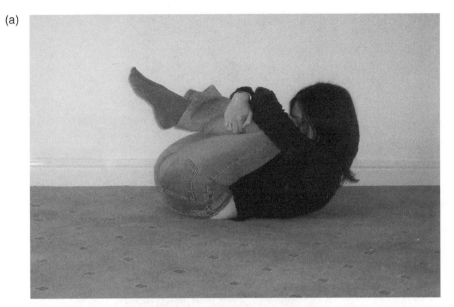

(b)

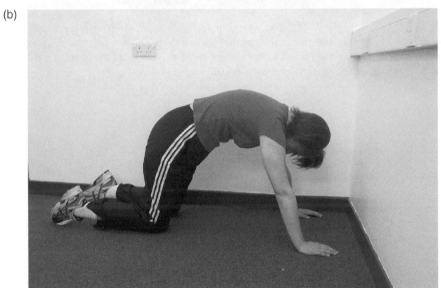

Figure 11.A6 Stretch for the small of the back. (a) Lying with both knees pulled up to the chest, grasp the knees with both arms and slowly bring up forehead towards knees. (b) An easier alternative: position yourself on the floor on all fours. Pull your stomach in towards your spine and round out your back from your tail bone to your neck. Hold for 15–30 s

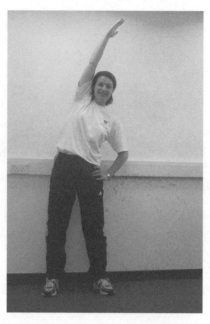

Figure 11.A7   Side stretch. Standing with your feet wide apart, stretch the right arm up and reach high and slightly over to one side, so that you are stretching just past the midline of your body. Hold for 15–30 s, then return to the upright position and repeat the stretch on the other side. Try not to let the trunk fall forwards or backwards

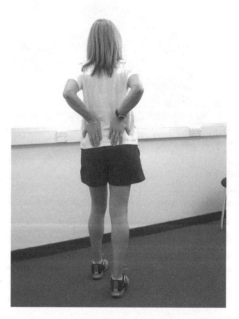

Figure 11.A8   Chest and shoulder stretch. Place both hands on the small of your back, keeping your elbows to the back, gently squeeze your elbows towards each other. Keep your head up and shoulders down and back. Hold for 15–30 s

(a)

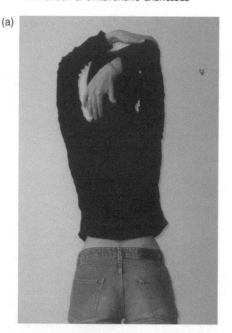

(b)

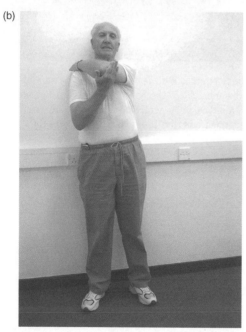

Figure 11.A9 Shoulder stretch. (a) Lift the right arm above the head, bend at the elbow and drop the right hand below the shoulder. Use the other hand to grasp the right elbow and ease it gently backwards to reach full stretch. Hold for 15–30 s and then slowly repeat with the other shoulder. (b) As an easier alternative, bring your right arm across in front of your body and pull gently with your left arm until you feel a stretch across your right shoulder. Hold for 15–30 s. Repeat with the other shoulder

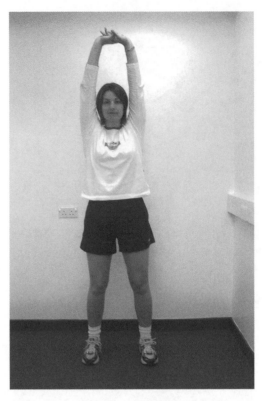

Figure 11.A10 Full body stretch. With feet comfortably apart, link fingers together and turn the palms upwards. Lift hands above the head so that the palms are facing towards the roof. Push the hands away from the body centre to achieve a full stretch. Hold for 15–30 s. This stretch can also be performed lying on the floor with the toes fully stretched

Appendix 2: Muscular Edurance Exercises

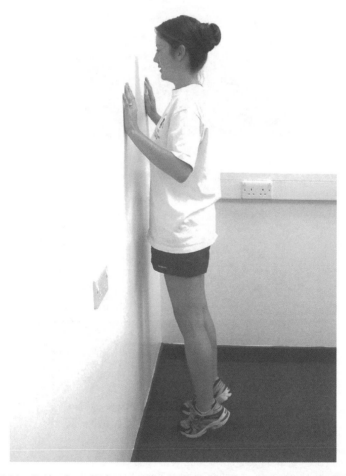

Figure 11.A11 Heel raises. Facing a wall, rest both hands on the wall at shoulder level for balance. Start with the feet flat on the floor. Then raise heels as high as possible whilst keeping the balls of your feet on the floor

(a)

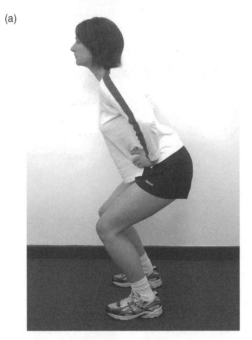

(b)

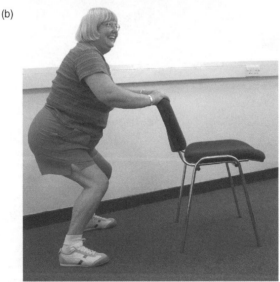

Figure 11.A12   Half Squat. (a) With feet shoulder-width apart and toes pointing forward, bend your knees and push your bottom out behind you. Keep your back straight. The hips should go no lower than the thighs being parallel with the floor. Keep your heels on the floor and knees behind your toes. If you look down from the squat position you should be able to see your toes. (b) To assist with balance, this exercise can be done with the aid of a chair

(a)

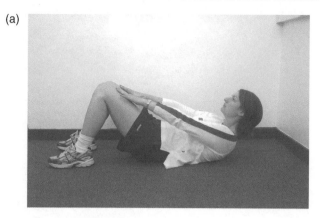

(b)

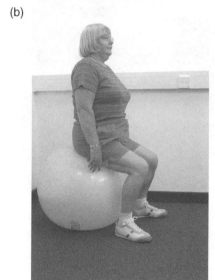 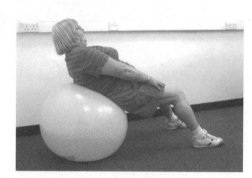

Figure 11.A13   Abdominal exercise. (a) Lying comfortably on your back with knees bent, breath out and push your lower back into the floor, then curl upwards. Keep your neck in line with your spine and eyes looking forward towards the ceiling. Run your hands up towards your knees as you curl. (b) Abdominal exercise can also be done using a physio ball. This alternative exercise is particularly good for people who have a heart condition as it keeps the head above heart level. Sit tall on the ball and walk the feet away from the ball, rolling the spine over the ball until the shoulder blades and mid back are in contact with the ball. Hold this position for a few seconds before tucking the chin in, curling the spine back and walking slowly back to the seated position

(a)

(b)

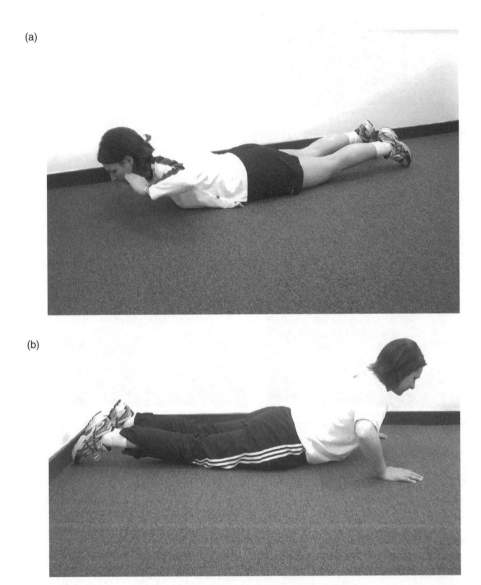

Figure 11.A14   Back raises. (a) Lying-face down with hands under the chin and elbows flexed, use the back muscles to raise the upper part of the body slowly from the ground. Hips and lower part of the body remain on the floor. Keep your eyes looking forwards towards the floor. (b) As an easier alternative, instead of having your hands at your chin, place them on the floor in line with the shoulders and use them to support the movement

(a)

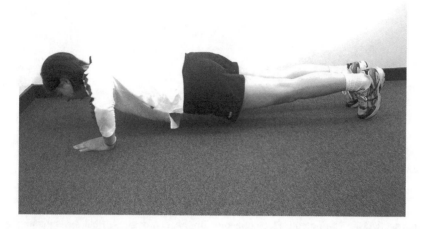

(b)

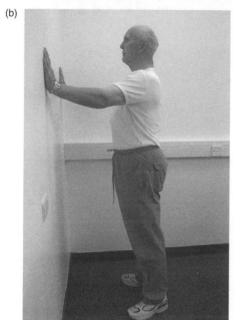 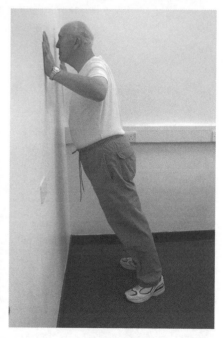

Figure 11.A15 Press up and wall press. This exercise can be performed against the wall (b), from the knees and hands or from the toes and hands (a). Hands are placed below the shoulders and the head kept in front of the hands. Elbows are straightened then bent. The back should be kept straight and the head in line with the spine

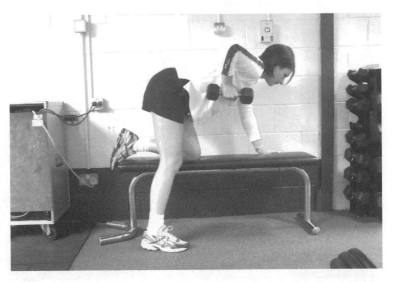

Figure 11.A16   Rowing pull. Place one knee on a bench or chair. Hold a weight in one hand and pull it up until it is in line with your chest, with your elbows pointing up to the ceiling. Keep your back straight

(a)   (b)

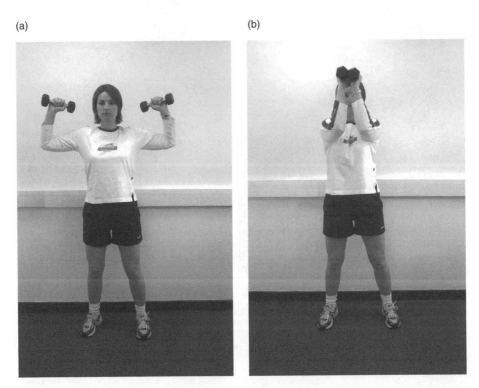

Figure 11.A17   Pec-dec. Keeping elbows at shoulder height, start with them out to the side (a) then bring elbows together (b). Return out to the sides

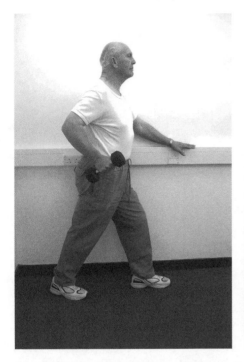 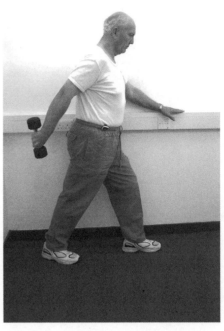

Figure 11.A18   Tricep extension. Using a small weight held at your hip, stand with one foot in front of the other. Move your arm from the bent position (90° angle) to a straightened position (180° angle). Keep the top half of the arm still and the shoulders relaxed

12

The Role of the Diabetes Team in Promoting Physical Activity

Dinesh Nagi and **Bill Burr**

12.1 Introduction

Modification of diet and physical activity is the cornerstone of the initial management plan of type 2 diabetes. In reality, however, many patients require oral agents or insulin to achieve satisfactory glycaemic control. It is also recognized that success in diabetes care depends to a large extent on patient self-care behaviours such as knowledge, attitude and motivation in influencing long-term outcomes.[1,2]

The benefits, risks, motivation, barriers and the type of physical activity which may be acceptable varies considerably among individuals. This variation is dependent upon many factors such as age, sex, ethnicity, associated medical conditions and socioeconomic and cultural influences, and perhaps other personal characteristics. It is accepted that, in subjects with type 1 diabetes, there are no proven benefits of exercise in improving glycaemic control and the main reasons for exercise are recreational or to achieve physical fitness. Individuals with type 1 diabetes who wish to participate actively in sports or exercise need adequate support from the diabetes teams. An intensive educational programme and materials need to be available for these individuals to educate them about the potential risks of physical activity and the precautions they need to take to exercise safely.

Therefore, for diabetes teams, the importance of physical activity and sport, especially in young people with type 1 diabetes, is related largely to the way in which the quest for good metabolic control can prove to be a barrier to their taking part in activities they would otherwise enjoy. It is hoped that the advice contained in earlier chapters (chapters 2, 5, 7 and 8) may help to avoid this. Those with type 1

Exercise and Sport in Diabetes, 2nd Edition   Edited by Dinesh Nagi
© 2005 John Wiley & Sons, Ltd.

diabetes may still share in the general health benefits which accrue to those taking regular exercise. It is worth remembering that inactive people who do *not* have diabetes have twice the risk of premature death and serious illness as those who keep active.[3]

In addition, sedentary living is now recognized to be the fourth primary risk factor for coronary heart disease behind hypertension, cholesterol and smoking.[4,5] People with type 1 diabetes have an increased risk of coronary artery disease, and those who keep active should expect to enjoy benefits in terms of reduced risk of cardiovascular disease, as well as the improved exercise capacity and psychological well-being associated with physical activity.[6]

In contrast, the health benefits of regular physical activity in type 2 diabetes have been clearly established, are evidence-based,[7] and were reviewed in detail in Chapter 6. They include improved metabolic control, reduced cardiovascular risks, reduced adiposity, increased physical fitness, improved psychological well-being and reduced cardiovascular mortality. It follows, then, that increased physical activity is a fundamental part of the treatment package for type 2 diabetes, and the diabetes team has a clear responsibility to promote and encourage this.

Our success in achieving the lifestyle changes necessary for good metabolic control in type 2 patients has been limited. The results of the recently published UK Prospective Diabetes Study confirm this in terms of weight control.[8] The conventionally treated group increased weight by approximately 5 kg during a median follow-up of 10 years, and the intensively treated group increased weight by about 10 kg, which is undesirable given the importance of weight loss for successful management of the condition. However, we must remember that the benefits of physical activity on glycaemic control are independent of weight loss.[9]

Most patients with type 2 diabetes take little or no physical activity, as shown in a large NHANES survey from USA.[10] In this survey, 31 per cent of people with diabetes reported no regular physical activity; another 38 per cent reported less than the currently recommended levels of physical activity. Lifestyle changes are never easy to achieve and sustain over a long period of time, but we must ask ourselves why patients are not managing to do what is required.

- Is it due to a failure to inform and educate patients about the benefits of regular physical exercise?

- Is it due to the inability of our patients to break down the barriers to physical activity in spite of adequate knowledge about the need to be more active?

- Is it due to a general lack of social, family and emotional support for these patients to help them to achieve and sustain an increase in physical activity?

- Is it due to associated co-morbidities?

- Is it due to a lack of motivation and personal commitment?

It is likely that all these factors combine to varying degrees in different patients. Strategies for dealing with these problems are dealt with later. It may also be relevant to consider as to how much time and effort is being spent promoting physical activity routinely in most diabetic clinics.

12.2 Educating the Diabetes Team

There is a need for all health professionals dealing with type 2 diabetes to understand the crucial role of increasing physical activity in treating the disease. We recently surveyed such professionals working in the UK. Most were aware of the benefits of physical activity, but spent very little time on physical activity assessment and education. A majority felt that the advice currently being offered is inadequate, unlikely to lead to lifestyle changes, and in need of improvement. The findings suggested that there is an awareness of the increasing importance of exercise in diabetes management, but that there may be a problem of identifying time, staff and facilities to deal properly with the subject.[11]

Historically, the make-up of specialist diabetes teams has been mainly influenced by the care requirements of patients with type 1 diabetes and its complications. This accounts for the inclusion of doctors, dieticians, specialist nurses and podiatrists in most diabetes teams. The care requirements of people with type 2 diabetes have usually had to be fitted into a pattern of care developed for insulin-treated patients. Unlike type 1 disease, type 2 diabetes is predominantly a lifestyle disease, and successful treatment requires adjustments of diet, weight and physical activity. Patients need to make these changes and to sustain them over many years, even though they may have few, if any, symptoms. To achieve this requires effective communication and educational skills as well as an ability to motivate. These attributes are not necessarily the same as those possessed by diabetologists, nurse specialists or dieticians, and this may partly explain our limited success in treating type 2 diabetes.

The National Service Framework (NSF) for Diabetes in England, UK has set the quality framework and the standards of care for people with diabetes.[12] It suggests that the needs of people with type 2 diabetes may be better served in primary care. It may be that members of the primary care team are better placed to take on this role. However, without appropriate education of health professionals, they may not appreciate the crucial importance of lifestyle changes in the management of diabetes. They should not, for instance, be too eager to introduce drug therapies such as sulfonylureas and insulin, which can encourage weight gain, without an adequate trial of lifestyle changes first.

12.3 Exercise Therapist as Part of the Team?

In addition to the fundamental deficiency of β-cell secretion in type 2 diabetes, there is a clear deficiency of physical activity. It follows, then that there is a need for a member of the diabetes team to have expert knowledge of this important intervention in the disease management. Such a person needs to be enthusiastic and possess knowledge about the benefits of physical activity. However, their ability to expend significant amounts of time is likely to be limited by other commitments. Therefore, a person with primary expertise in exercise, who understands the importance of physical activity in the treatment of diabetes, might have a role in this area.

We believe that an exercise therapist would be able to work with other members of the diabetes team to produce physical activity programmes appropriate for a patient's health needs. He or she should also be able to lead group activity programmes – which seem to be particularly successful with female patients – and could supervise exercise sessions in a gym, physiotherapy department or diabetes centre; such sessions at the beginning of a weight loss programme have been shown to improve success rates.[13] Group sessions help to demonstrate to people the kind of activities and aerobic exercises they can perform safely, and give an opportunity for a person to meet others who are in a similar situation. In a broader context, the exercise therapist should be able to educate other groups dealing with diabetes care about the most effective ways of motivating and guiding patients to take more exercise.

Given the anticipated changes in the care provision to patients with diabetes as discussed above, the specialist exercise therapist should or could be based in primary care. It is important that there should be close working relationships with both primary and specialist diabetes teams, in order to promote any educational activity.

12.4 Assessment of Patients

Every patient needs full evaluation before commencing exercise. This will include a medical examination as well as an assessment of current levels of physical activity, and attitudes to exercise. These can be easily remembered by mnemonic, the ABCDEF of physical activity promotion.

The medical (generally done by a physician) examination should include:

1. *Assessment*

   (a) Medical history:

   - details of diabetes specific history – current treatment, symptoms related to hyper- or hypoglycaemia, and episodes of diabetic keto acidosis (DKA);

   - symptoms and treatment of chronic complications of diabetes such as laser treatment, foot problems;

   - cardiac history of angina, previous heart attacks, coronars artery bypass graft, angioplasty, results of an exercise stress test if performed, history of palpitation or tachycardia;

- hypertension;
- family history of ischaemic heart disease or sudden death;
- history of previous stroke or transient ischaemic attacks;
- previous musculoskeletal injuries;
- history of smoking and alcohol intake.

(b) Physical examination:

- anthropometry;
- full cardiological assessment – pulse rate, peripheral pulses, blood pressure, heart sound, any murmurs, any signs of congestive cardiac failure;
- examinations for complications of diabetes, i.e. retinopathy, neuropathy;
- detailed foot examination for deformity, pressure areas, arthritis, etc.

(c) Biochemical investigations:

- full blood count, urea/creatinine, lipids, thyroid function test, HbA1c, urine for albumin.

(d) Cardiac investigations:

- resting echocardiogram in all over 35 years of age;
- other investigation, such as cardiac echocardiogram or exercise stress testing, should only be performed when clinically indicated.

(e) Risk assessment for macro vascular disease:

- should be performed depending upon history, physical examination and the results of investigations.

(f) Assessment in relation to physical activity (member of diabetes team interested in exercise):

- current levels of physical activity;
- knowledge about the benefits and risks of physical activity;
- personal attitudes and barriers to physical activity;
- psychosocial and economic factors as these clearly influence the choice and type of physical activity.

2. *Behaviour modification* in relation to physical activity/modes of exercise:

   - tips for safe activities;

   - self-monitoring through exercise diaries;

   - target setting (frequency, duration, weight targets in obese);

   - continued contact, supervision, motivation, confidence building;

   - the key aim is to expend calories, and typical activities include walking, cycling, jogging, swimming and sports activities (badminton, tennis etc.).

3. *Commitment to change* – physical activity behaviour is a major undertaking and therefore will require careful planning on the part of the patient and the health professional. Once exercise has commenced, its success is crucial for building confidence, which in turn helps to develop a stronger attitude and commitment with less reliance on external support. However, even the most committed individuals who exercise on a regular basis require some degree of support and recognition.

4. *Decision-making and goal setting* – this can be helped by the use of 'decision balance sheets', which have been shown to increase commitment to behaviour change, particularly at the outset.[14] This would include setting an initial feasible and easily achievable target with a high likelihood of success. Over a period of time the patient can work in close collaboration with the health professional in charge of exercise promotion to review and change targets. This clearly will help to optimize the benefits of an exercise programme and help develop a professional relationship and mutual trust. As time passes and the patient gains more confidence and is successful in achieving these targets, this will reduce the continual need for frequent contact due to self-sufficiency.

5. *Encouragement and support* are required particularly at the outset and can take various forms. They are needed in some shape or form for all wishing to be physically active but particularly those in action or ready for action. It may be the provision of information, listening to the difficulties or any other considerations from the patient regarding their experiences. Patients like recognition for their achievements and the health professional may become an exercise mentor for these patients.

6. *Formulation of physical activity programme* – Most diabetes clinics do not at present allocate a specific place for education about physical activity in their programmes for people with type 2 diabetes. Our preliminary observations suggest that, by adopting focused advice regarding physical activity, it may be possible to significantly influence the levels of self-reported physical activity, compared with those given routine advice.[15] To be successful, we will also have to adopt innovative methods for this behaviour modification.

12.5 The Exercise Prescription

For many people with diabetes, especially those with type 2 disease and those starting to exercise, even moderate exercise would be a challenge. It is important to get over the message that every little helps. The daily exercise target can be built up in small parcels of activity, so it is vital to stress the importance of seemingly trivial activities such as avoiding the use of lifts and escalators, parking a little further from the supermarket, getting off at a bus stop which is not the nearest, etc. The exercise prescription for health improvement has already been stated in earlier chapters, but can be summarized as being equivalent to 30 min of moderate physical exertion (such as very brisk 4 mph walking), on five or six days a week. If the exertion is of lesser or greater intensity, then it should be continued for longer or shorter periods, as suggested in Table 12.1. General advice about the safety of exercise and the necessary precautions to avoid problems has been given in previous chapters (Chapters 2, 6 and 11). The watchword for those starting to exercise is to *start low and go slow* – begin with small increases compared with current activity and build up gradually. Any untoward symptoms should be reported to medical advisers.

We feel that most patients with diabetes can increase their physical activity levels, with the type of activity being determined by an individual's personal preference, current lifestyle and any physical limitations and complications which

Table 12.1 The exercise prescription: recommended examples of moderate physical activity

30 minutes

- Walking very briskly on flat (2 miles, 4 mph), or carrying 25 lb load at 3 mph
- Gardening – weeding, mowing lawn (power mower), raking lawn
- Home – sweeping up, washing and waxing car, painting or plastering, washing windows
- Cycling leisurely (10 mph – 5 miles in 30 min)
- Dancing – ballroom
- Golf – using trolley for clubs
- Volleyball
- Badminton – doubles
- Horse riding

20 minutes

- Walking upstairs, back-packing, mountain walking
- Running (5 mph)
- Swimming (slow crawl, 50 yards min^{-1})
- Mowing lawn (hand mower)
- Tennis (singles)
- Basketball
- Cycling, moderate effort (12–14 mph)
- Activities to be performed ideally five or six times per week

Adapted from Ainsworth *et al.*[20]

may exist. The exercise prescription needs to be individualized and to achieve this detailed knowledge of a person's diabetes, lifestyle and beliefs about physical activity is very important. This enables the members of the diabetes team, in collaboration with the patient and his/her family, to discuss and formulate a structured programme of physical activity to optimize the health gains of exercise with minimal risk.

12.6   Patient Education

The main problem in promoting physical activity to people with newly diagnosed type 2 diabetes is their long-standing sedentary lifestyle.[10] Education regarding the benefits of physical activity should become a vital part in the management of type 2 diabetes. To do this at the time of initial diagnosis may be useful as the motivation for a behaviour change is at its highest. Furthermore, adopting physical activity is also a positive health behaviour change in contrast to many negative associations which go with the diagnosis of diabetes, such as restrictions on favourite foods, alcohol and smoking.

In the UK, the Health Education Council produces materials for exercise promotion for use by community and health professionals, but these are not specifically targeted to the problems of people with diabetes.[15] In promoting exercise and managing weight loss, graphs may be useful which show, for instance, the increased longevity associated with weight loss in newly diagnosed type 2 patients (Figure 12.1). More resource materials need to be available to

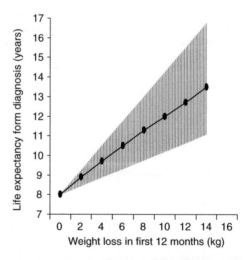

Figure 12.1   Life expectancy in patients with type 2 diabetes (body mass index >26 kg m^{-2}) in relation to weight loss in the first year of treatment. The shaded area represents the 95% confidence intervals. Adapted from Lean *et al.*,[21] by permission

Table 12.2   Potential health benefits of 10 kg weight loss in a patient weighing 100 kg

Mortality

- 20–25% fall in total mortality
- 30–40% fall in diabetes-related deaths
- 40–50% fall in obesity-related cancer deaths

Blood pressure

- Fall of approximately 10 mmHg in systolic/diastolic

Diabetes

- >50% reduction in risk of developing diabetes
- 30–50% fall in fasting glucose
- 15% fall in HbAlc

Lipids

- 10% fall in total cholesterol
- 15% fall in LDL cholesterol
- 30% fall in triglycerides
- 8% increase in HDL cholesterol

Reprinted from Jung,[22] 1997, by permission of Oxford University Press.

diabetes teams to assist them in their efforts to promote physical activity in patients, particularly those with type 2 disease.

Other information, on benefits of weight loss in terms of reduced risk of diabetes, improved diabetes control, lower blood pressure and lipid levels, and improved survival (Table 12.2), may be useful for the education of health professionals and, with suitable adaptation, for education of patients. Material produced primarily to highlight the benefits of weight loss may be used while discussing the advantages of physical activity, since increased activity has been shown to maintain weight loss. We need a better selection of eye-catching and persuasive material to highlight the benefits of physical activity.

12.7   Motivating Patients and Changing Behaviour

When attempting to motivate patients towards becoming more active, it is worth noting that the very word 'exercise' has strong negative associations for the type of person we are usually trying to encourage. In many people's minds it is linked to visions of youth and athletic endeavour, and it is important that we take care not to foster this notion by our choice of words. For this reason we deliberately choose to talk about 'physical activity', rather than 'exercise' or 'sport'.

In the previous chapter the 'stages of change' model was detailed as an approach to achieving lifestyle alterations. Briefly, according to this model, it is necessary to establish the patient's attitude to increasing physical activity before deciding on the approach to take. Some will have given the idea no thought at all, consider it to be a waste of time or unimportant, and have no intention of starting to exercise (pre-contemplators). Others may have accepted that they should be taking more exercise, but will have not yet made any changes (contemplators), while some will actually be trying to do more (action), and yet others may have tried and failed (relapse). Finally, there will be some who have been successful in making change but need support to sustain this change. Having established where the patient lies on the spectrum of stages of change, it is possible to derive appropriate strategies to help them to move from one stage to another. This would ensure that interventions are matched to the patient's state of mind, and therefore most likely to meet with success.

Patients are likely to need a great deal of encouragement and support, especially in the early stages when they are at the stage of 'action' or are ready for action. Encouragement may take the form of providing information, recounting difficulties encountered by others, or lending a sympathetic ear to problems which the patient may be having. Even the most committed individuals who exercise on a regular basis need some recognition and support from time to time.

Tackling barriers to physical activity

These may be physical or psychological. The physical barriers are probably easier to recognize, and have to be allowed for in developing a safe exercise plan. However, it is also important to keep in mind the various psychological factors which can lead to negative attitudes, and experiences which are likely to prevent patients from exercising also need to be addressed.

- 'Not being a sporty type' is the most common reason given by middle-aged or older people for not taking exercise.[16] It must be linked to a lack of knowledge about the relatively low levels of physical activity required in order to benefit health, and should therefore be relatively easy to overcome during initial education (see Table 12.1).

- Embarrassment about physique is a major problem in dealing with the obese type 2 patients, especially females. It can be a complete barrier to them taking part in activities such as swimming, which in other respects is an ideal activity for these patients. It may sometimes be dealt with successfully in group activities, where others have the same problems, so that group aerobic or swimming sessions can help to break down initial embarrassment. Educational materials which feature overweight people in a favourable manner can also be very helpful in boosting confidence to allow such patients to start exercising.

- Self-confidence – obese and inactive people are likely to have low levels of self-esteem, and the diagnosis of diabetes is probably going to reduce this still further. These people are very likely to have negative attitudes to their body image, and to the idea of taking exercise. The fact that control of diabetes requires that the issues of weight and inactivity are confronted is almost certainly going to provoke even more negative responses. The health professional needs to be sensitive to the vulnerable state of the newly diagnosed type 2 patient. Goals in relation to both exercise and diet need to be realistic, to ensure that the patient is capable of achieving them. In this way confidence can progressively be built up as activity increases. At the same time, the professional needs to be generous with praise to promote confidence-building exercise.

Setting goals which are achievable

It has been suggested that the use of 'decision balance sheets' (Table 12.3), may increase commitment for a behaviour change, particularly at the outset.[17] This

Table 12.3. Exercise decision balance sheet

Walking back to health: your personal decision balance sheet			

Target behaviour

Taking three 30 min lunch-time walks on Monday, Wednesday and Friday this week.

Reasons for exercising	Impact	Reasons against exercising	Impact
I know it will make me feel better	☐	I can't seem to find the time	☐
It will help me manage my weight	☐	I don't really know what I have to do	☐
I enjoy getting out of the house	☐	I feel embarrassed about exercise	☐
It makes me feel fitter and in control	☐	I feel guilty about taking the time	☐
It is something positive I can do	☐	I find it painful	☐
I want to show others that I can do it	☐	There is nowhere safe to exercise	☐
Other	☐	Other	☐
Other	☐	Other	☐
Total positive impact	☐	Total negative impact	☐

Strategies for improvement

Add in more positive reasons or make existing ones more powerful, e.g. *I enjoy walking as it makes me spend time with my friends*

Eliminate or reduce the reasons against, e.g. *I have talked about walking for health with my family and they want to help me find some personal time. I now feel supported and less guilty*

Patients should be encouraged to generate their own lists of positive and negative factors

Adapted from reference by Fox,[18] by permission.

would include setting an initial feasible and easily achievable target with high likelihood of success. For example, this might involve a decision (as illustrated) to walk three days a week. Potential benefits and negatives are listed and given values to reflect their relative importance to the patient. Over a period of time the patient can work with the health professional in charge of exercise promotion to review and change targets, and to maximize benefits and reduce the impact of negative factors.[18] This goal-setting exercise is a useful way of establishing new exercise habits, and this can be reinforced if the patient also keeps an activity record that can be used to build on successes and to help formulate new targets. The initial aim is to build up the frequency of exercise, followed by exercise duration and then intensity.

The following case histories illustrate some of the benefits of increased physical activity in patients with type 2 diabetes. We have included them in the hope that this will encourage colleagues to adopt similar strategies for dealing with the lifestyle problems of such patients.

Case history 1

A 46-year-old man had been diagnosed as having type 2 diabetes at the age of 31 and followed up at another hospital. He was seen at the Edna Coates Diabetes Centre in August 1995. He had no symptoms of hyperglycaemia and had noticed that his blood sugars at home had been running 'high'. He was a non-smoker and drank 16 units of alcohol a week. His medication was metformin 850 mg three times daily and glibenclamide 5 mg twice daily. His weight was 93.1 kg, body mass index 27, blood pressure 131/84 mmHg, HbA1c 10.6 per cent (3.1–5.0).

The patient was commenced on insulin treatment, and in July 1996 he weighed 104.6 kg, his HbA1c was 5.7 per cent, and he was taking 45 units of Humulin I twice daily. He had gained 11.6 kg, although there had also been a dramatic improvement in his diabetic control. However, in November 1996, his control had slipped back: HbA1c 7.3 per cent and weight 106 kg. As he was concerned about weight gain, and his diabetic control had worsened, he was advised to take up regular physical activity. Six months later, he had managed to reduce his insulin by a total of 20 units/day and his HbA1c had improved to 5.8 per cent. He converted his garage into a mini-gym and exercised for 60 min/day 3–4 days a week. In addition to reducing his total dose of insulin by about 25 per cent, his diabetic control had improved. The patient felt 'excellent' and physically fit, with improved quality of life.

Case history 2

A 53-year-old woman had been found to have type 2 diabetes in May 1991, and was markedly symptomatic. She weighed 134 kg (body mass index 50.3), and was commenced on a diet and metformin 500 mg three times daily. In January 1992, she weighed 125 kg, had no glycosuria and was lost to follow-up (she was worried that she had not lost enough weight and would be 'told off'). She was seen again at the diabetes centre in June 1997 because she was again symptomatic, and surprisingly weighed 99 kg, body mass index 37, HbA1c 8.8 per cent. In August 1997 she weighed 93.7 kg and was taking metformin 850 mg three times daily. In addition, she had started floor exercises, 20 min daily, walked for 90 min most days of the week, and took stairs to her office (situated on the 11th floor). She had instituted a strict programme of diet and exercise and in 12 months had lost nearly 21 kg, while her glycaemic control had improved slightly, with an HbA1c of 8.3 per cent.

There are two messages from this case. First, she had done well first time around, having lost about 6 per cent of total body weight, and should have been congratulated on her achievements. Second, building a programme of exercise that fits into one's lifestyle is likely to be sustained in the long run.

Case history 3

A 49-year-old male non-obese subject with type 2 diabetes presented in October 1995 with osmotic symptoms, and was commenced on treatment with diet and gliclazide 80 mg once daily. His HbA1c was 9.9 per cent, and gliclazide was increased to 80 mg twice daily. In April 1996, he was seen at the diabetes centre and had a body mass index of 25, 5 per cent glycosuria and HbA1c 7.4 per cent. Metformin was added at 500 mg three times daily. In July 1996, his glycaemic control had deteriorated further and HbA1c had risen to 9.0 per cent. He was advised to take regular physical activity, and 6 months later had an HbA1c of 6.8 per cent. He was now walking for 30 min during his lunch break and 60 min in the evening.

In summary:

- All subjects with type 2 diabetes should be assessed for their leisure time and occupational activity.

- They should be screened for complications of diabetes before starting a formal exercise programme.

- Those who currently take little or no exercise but are ready for action should be given individualized advice to encourage increased activity.

- All patients with type 2 diabetes should have education regarding exercise, and this should form an essential part of ongoing education.

- Diabetes teams should take a lead role in developing information leaflets and highlighting the health benefits of exercise.

12.8 Conclusions

There is good evidence that increased physical activity leads to a number of health benefits, which are particularly important in the treatment and prevention of type 2 diabetes. Diabetes teams need to provide full information about the role of inactivity in the causation of type 2 diabetes, and the fact that successful treatment requires an increase in physical activity. They also need to be able to motivate patients to be more active, and to provide long-term support to maintain behaviour change. Diabetes teams need to give exercise promotion at least equal importance to advice concerning diet and disease monitoring. However, this is likely to require extra resources as well as a great deal of commitment from members of the diabetes team. Whatever programmes we design and implement to promote physical activity will have to be evaluated to determine their cost-effectiveness in the overall management of type 2 diabetes.[19]

References

1. Clement S. Diabetes self-management education. *Diabetes Care* 1995; **18**: 1204–1214.
2. Glasgow RE, Ruggiero L, Eakin EG, Dryfoos JM, Chobarian I. Diabetes self-management. *Diabetes Care* 1997; **4**: 568–576.
3. Killoran AJ, Fentem P, Casperson C (eds). *Moving On: International Perspectives on Promoting Physical Activity.* London: Health Education Authority, 1994.
4. Powell KE, Thompson PD, Casperson CJ, Ford ES. Physical activity and the incidence of coronary heart disease. *A Rev Public Health* 1987; **8**: 253–287.
5. Berlin JA, Colditz GA. A meta-analysis of physical activity in the prevention of coronary heart disease. *Am J Epidemiol* 1990; **132**: 612–628.
6. Blair SN, Hardman A. Special issue: physical activity, health and well- being – an international consensus conference. *Res Q Exerc Sport* 1995; **66**(4).
7. American Diabetes Association. Exercise and NIDDM (Technical Review). *Diabetes Care* 1990; **13**: 785–789.
8. United Kingdom Prospective Diabetes Study Group. UK Prospective Diabetes Study 33: intensive blood glucose control with sulphonylureas or insulin compared with conventional treatment and risk of complications in patients with type 2 diabetes. *Lancet* 1998; **352**: 837–853.
9. Boule NG, Haddad E, Kenny GP, Wells GA, Sigal RJ. Effects of exercise on glycaemic control and body mass in type 2 diabetes mellitus. A meta-analysis of controlled clinical trials. *JAMA* 2001; **286**: 1218–1227.
10. Nelson K, Gayle R, Boyko E. Diet and exercise among adults with type 2 diabetes. Findings form the Third National Health and Nutrition Examination Survey (NHANES III). *Diabetes Care* 2002; **25**: 1722–1728.
11. Berlanga F, Wareham N, Burr WA, Nagi DK. Pyscial activity in type 2 diabetes: current case patterns: a survey of diabetes health professionals. *Pract Diabet Int* 2000; **17**: 60–61.
12. The National Service Framework for Diabetes, 2002; www.doh.gov.uk/nsf/diabetes/research
13. Craighead LW, Blum MD. Supervised exercise in behavioural treatment for moderate obesity. *Behav Ther* 1989; **20**: 49–59.

14. Wankel LM. Decision-making and social support strategies for increasing exercise involvement. *J Cardiac Rehabil* 1984; **4**: 124–135.
15. Berlanga F, Wareham N, Burr WA, Nagi DK. Does a 'focused' advice to increase physical activity work in patients with newly diagnosed type 2 diabetes? *Diab Med* 1998 (suppl. 1): S2.
16. Health Education Authority. *A Guide to Physical Activity Promotion in Primary Care in England*. London: Health Education Authority, 1996.
17. Health Education Authority and Sports Council. *Allied Dunbar National Fitness Survey: Main Findings*. London: Health Education Authority, 1992.
18. Fox KR. Promoting physical activity in people with diabetes. *Pract Diabet Int* 1998; **15**: 146–150.
19. Graber Al, Christman BG, Alogna MT, Davidson JK. Evaluation of diabetes patient education programme. *Diabetes* 1977; **26**: 61–64.
20. Ainsworth BE, Haskell WL, Leon AS *et al.* Compendium of physical activities: classification of energy costs of human activities. *Med Sci Sports Exerc* 1993; **25**: 71–80.
21. Lean ME, Powrie JK, Anderson AS, Garthwaite PH. Obesity, weight loss and prognosis in type 2 diabetes. *Diab Med* 1990; **7**: 228–233.
22. Jung RT. Obesity as a disease. *Br Med Bull* 1997; **53**: 307–321.

Index

Note: page numbers in *italics* refer to figures and tables.

Exercise and Sport in Diabetes, 2nd Edition Edited by Dinesh Nagi
© 2005 John Wiley & Sons, Ltd.

Index compiled by Jill Halliday